HOPE
is my
Wingman

Michael Antcliffe

Split Tree Publishing
Thunder Bay, Ontario, Canada

HOPE IS MY WINGMAN
was originally published in 2012 as
You'll Never Guess Who's Dying From Cancer

This book may be ordered at a highly discounted price by registered non-profit associations related to cancer awareness, patient care, or research by contacting the publisher at *www.splittreepublishing.com/cancercare*.

More information about Michael and his fundraising initiative can be found at *www.michaelantcliffe.com* or *www.facebook.com/HopeismyWingman*

Printed in the United States of America.

DEDICATION

First and foremost, I must dedicate this book to my mother, Mary. All that is good about me, including any good I may manage to do, is credited to this amazing woman and the caring, loving manner in which she raised my siblings and me.

This book is also dedicated to my father, Alan, because without the strength and courage he taught me, I surely would have faltered on this path long ago.

Thank you to the thousands of people who have shown the courage to support me and have volunteered to lose a friend to cancer. They may not yet fully understand the courage they have shown, but in time I believe they will. It is my sincere hope that they have marked a path for thousands more to follow.

This book is dedicated to the countless many who have walked their own paths with cancer, for those who are walking that path right now, and for the many we hope to spare with our collective efforts. Cancer comes in many horrific forms and it does not discriminate whom it touches or the lives it tears apart.

This book is finally dedicated to all those who choose to fight, everyone who chooses to draw a line in the sand and demand an end to this once invincible menace in our lifetime, because that's what we are capable of.

Russel Richard Ciotucha
September 20th 1978 – September 24th 2010

There is a Reaper whose name is Death,
And, with his sickle keen,
He reaps the bearded grain at a breath,
And the flowers that grew between.

~ Henry Wadsworth Longfellow

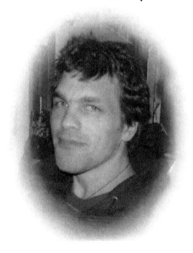

ACKNOWLEDGMENTS

First and foremost, I would like to thank Stacey Voss; without her, this endeavour would not have been possible. I would also like to thank Kevin Chlebovec for working so closely with her, and my friend Josh Fitzgerald for helping with pictures.

Sincere appreciation to those who contributed their own thoughts, words and photos: Anne Raynor, Ames Lazer, Christine Bertoldo, Janice Kelly, Kathy, Sean Collis, Teri Antcliffe, and Hayley McLeod.

My thanks for media support from Lisa Laco, Mark Tannahill, and Russel MacKenzie.

Deepest thanks to the Thunder Bay Regional Health Science Centre and Princess Margaret Hospital for their tireless work and assistance in keeping me alive for so long.

Last, but certainly not least, I would like to show my love for my family, friends, and Facebook supporters.

FOREWORD

This is actually the third time I've written a foreword for Michael's book. The first foreword sounds awkward to me now. I had only met Michael in person a handful of times when I wrote the first one and, to be honest, I was still a little in awe of the guy. The second foreword was written in grief, after I had spent a lot of time with Michael and he had somehow crept into my heart and become one of my dearest friends.

This time I want to give you some insight into the Michael I knew. I didn't know the Michael who existed before he was told that his life was ending. That man is a bit of a mystery to me, but from the stories I've heard, he really didn't change all that drastically.

Many of my stories with Michael take place in my car. We did a lot of driving, whether it was running down to the border to pick up books, driving to appointments, or just going to get ice cream. Whenever I sit in the passenger seat of my car now, I picture the way he would get in and settle himself, put his things in the glove compartment, adjust the seat, and generally make himself as comfortable as possible.

My favourite story is from the day I took Michael and his photographer friend, Josh, down to pick up our first full shipment of books before the big launch. Michael had his hoodie and sunglasses on, shading his eyes and skin from the negative side effects the sun inflicted on him as a result of the miraculous medication he was currently taking. Having never had a problem at the border before, I didn't expect what happened next. The

American border guards appeared very tense as they asked us to come inside and one followed our car on foot as I parked and walked behind us with his hand on his gun as we went inside.

I was really confused about what was happening. I had never been in trouble before and I made a joke to Michael that maybe the reason they were pulling us in was because he still had his sunglasses on. He quipped, "I never take them off." The border guard barked, "You'll take them off when I tell you to take them off." The tone of his voice really brought home the seriousness of our situation. Up until that point, I had thought it was maybe just some random check.

When we got inside, the guard took Michael down to the end of the counter. He frisked him and had him empty his pockets. The guard asked him a series of questions, his voice still holding the same abrupt tone, until he asked Michael what he did for a living. Michael answered that he was on disability. The guard almost sneered as he asked him what was wrong with him. When Michael answered that he had cancer, you could see the body language of the guard change. I could see his eyes look at Michael's appearance with a new point of view. Instead of seeing a skinny drug-dealer in a hoodie and shades, he now saw the fragile, bald man who was fighting for his life.

The guard quickly finished up with Mike and half-heartedly called me up. I emptied my pockets and out came an engraved rock I had grabbed before I left home, intending to give it to Michael.

"Can I give this to him?" I asked the guard, motioning toward Mike, "I brought it for him."

The guard almost seemed to shrink visibly as he read the word Hope engraved on the stone. I handed it to Mike. "I brought this for you, since you lost your rock of Courage. I figured you could use a rock of Hope."

The guard never even took a second glance at Josh. He left the room and another guard told us we could leave.

I was angry about the experience for a few days, until I really thought about it. The guard was just doing his job. At least he was human enough to let go of the tough guy facade when he realized that Michael was not the thug that he had originally taken him to be.

During another trip to the border, I had a major issue with my stomach. I pulled over to the side of the road, and threw up, in extreme pain. I knew I couldn't drive the 45 minutes home. Luckily, Mike was having a good day and wasn't on the heavy painkillers. I decided to let him try and drive.

I remember leaning over the dash, looking over at Michael, trying to find a position where my stomach wasn't stabbing me with pain. He had such a look of pure joy on his face. He glanced over at me guiltily and apologized. He explained that he hadn't driven since Christmas and hadn't thought that he'd ever have the chance to drive a car again. Honestly, it made the pain worth it.

We made it safely back to the city. He drove like a pro, a small smile on his face the whole time.

Michael took joy in the little things and cared deeply about the people in his life. He never wanted to be a burden on anyone and was the most stubborn man I have ever met. His sense of humour was exceeded only by his compassion.

This book consists of notes and wall posts that Michael posted on Facebook, combined with some heartfelt notes written by some of the people he affected both in real life and online. It was originally published by Michael, Kevin, and me in April 2012 to help with Michael's fundraising efforts. Michael inspired Kevin and me to start a publishing company, Split Tree Publishing. Our very first publication is Michael's book and we are very proud of the fact that 90% of Net Profits from this book will be going to the Canadian Cancer Society. The other 10% will be used for marketing. We will do everything that we can to help Michael reach his goal of raising $1,000,000.00 to help people fighting cancer.

For those of you reading Michael's words for the first time, I ask you to listen to his message. Talk to your neighbours, tell your friends and family that you love them at every opportunity, pet strange dogs, and never, ever give up hope. Not every battle is won in the way we want or expect, but we can turn the result into the most positive experience it can be. And, by the way, I want you to ask yourself at the end, how do you feel about owing Michael ten bucks?

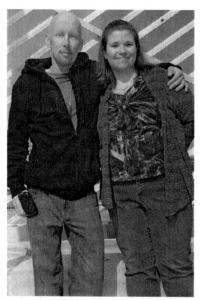

Michael and Stacey - March 22, 2012
Photo Courtesy of Josh Fitzgerald

YOU'LL NEVER GUESS WHO'S DYING FROM CANCER
THURSDAY, APRIL 21, 2011 AT 12:49 AM

You'll never guess who's dying from cancer. Gather 'round children, take a knee, and let me tell you a story. I am in the twelfth round of a fight that began three years ago. My opponent has quite an impressive record. The truth, which I now find myself at peace with, is that I'm going to lose. This is not the cancer I fought three years ago. This isn't even the cancer I fought three months or three weeks ago. For all of you, this is going to happen someday, but for me this is happening right now. I need your help to achieve something special. I need each of you to owe me ten bucks after I die, and I need you to ask all of your Facebook friends to do the same. I wanna raise a million dollars to provide care and comfort for other people in my position.

I don't know how long this fight will last, but I damned well know it has started. I'm certain the ride will be wild and filled with bad jokes (mostly mine). In the end, the only thing that I can promise is that I'll let you know how this turns out. Honestly, right now I'm somewhere between not keeping the receipts for anything and still looking both ways before crossing the street. Walk a few steps with me and volunteer to have a friend who is going to be taken by cancer. Take the time, the precious time, to compose a simple message to all of your other Facebook friends. Tell them they will never guess who's dying from cancer and tell them that I'm accepting all friends on Facebook, so long as they pony up with the dough when I die. Don't just click once and forget. We're both

1

working on the honour system here.

If this works, I will have truly found a way to be rich in friends. The more friends I get, the more comfort and peace we can all take part in providing. I promise to speak to you from this day to my last.

My good friend, Nicole, will cash the cheque. I'll be there to pick up the bill. Oh come on, that one's funny for sure. I need your help. Let's all play our part in this. Ask your friends to read this. Tell them you have a friend who's dying from cancer. My name is Michael Antcliffe and I want you to be my friend.

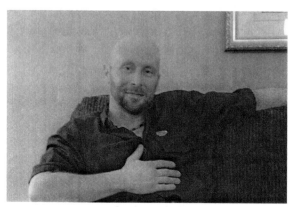

Michael Antcliffe
Photo Courtesy of Teri Antcliffe

GOOD MORNING
THURSDAY, APRIL 21, 2011 AT 1:09 PM

I awoke this morning to well-wishes, tales from the heart, and some great new friends to draw strength from. Thanks both to those I knew yesterday and to the new friends I find today for all of the encouragement and support. This feels good. I'm already wondering about tomorrow. Come on guys, forward my challenge. I want all of your Facebook friends. My burden feels smaller already because of you guys today. Think of the weight our collective shoulders could lift tomorrow.

IF YOU WERE EXPECTING A MILLION FRIENDS THIS MORNING, I THINK I KNOW EXACTLY WHO IS TO BLAME . . .
FRIDAY, APRIL 22, 2011 AT 6:12 PM

It's my fault, but not in the martyr or poster-boy sense. Let's say it's as much my fault as it is all of yours (newbies excluded). I hold myself as the worst example, far worse than any of you I may be about to offend.

Cancer took my own cousin not long ago. You know what I did? Sweet bugger all. Even worse, I looked away. I saw a member of my own bloodline suffering and I did not possess the courage to even place my hand on his chest to comfort him. I didn't come running when it looked like he needed me: I hid. I respected the strength of this man, but fear of my own place in such battles kept me silent and scared. I even showed the hypocrisy to post a request on his profile asking for courage and friends. I didn't do it purposefully to make this point but because I was scared out of my mind. As my cousin showed his courage, I showed up when requested by a braver family member. I cried or hugged someone when it felt appropriate. I placed my arm around his mother and offered comfort, a comfort that I now realize I did not possess the humility to offer him. Cancer is a harsh and unrelenting teacher; humility is one of its lessons. The evil of the indifference of good men makes me guilty as charged.

Meaningful interaction is lost in today's world. We barely even look at what makes up our own perspective, much less someone else's. Watch people walk down the street, watch them bump into real, potential friends while they text their electronic ones. I'm not a bad person and neither are you. But there are people on my original friends list that haven't so much as sent me a smiley face. I'm not their poster boy. I'm the guy they ran with in fields, met on the wrestling mat, and studied with in high school or university. We had sleepovers and hunted together. This isn't a milk carton situation. *You know me.* Until we all take a step back towards meaningful human interaction, I sure as hell don't deserve to raise any friends or money. So take the day off, stop caring about the goal, and enjoy the process. If, at the end of this, I only have the friends who have read this far, I will storm Hell's Gate with you. If, at the end of this, we have only afforded better coffee for cancer treatment waiting rooms (trust me, it's needed) then we should be proud. We interacted in a meaningful way, we peeled away a few layers of fear and discomfort, and we did more than *re-post* our feelings. Forget about the ten bucks you owe me. Go find that Facebook friend on your list that you've never spoken to. Let's not BS each other . . . we all have them. Ask them how they are doing. No answer . . . ask again! Then actively listen to their response. If you're not careful, you will find yourself immersed in a process that feels stranger to you than simply running through the motions of life. I'd appreciate it if you would tell them about me, but I think I'd understand if you don't.

And just to gently drive this point home (Hammer of Thor) my person for the day is my Aunt Teri. She messaged me yesterday. She said, "Three years, just finding out now, I feel sick." I knew immediately how she felt. I could see the tears in her eyes. We lived three blocks from one another at one point and I have not had the courage to reach out to her for help. I will be back in Thunder Bay on Sunday and I will find her by Monday. Auntie Teri, I love you; I don't want you to have that sick feeling. You and I will interact meaningfully with our time, we will have a humble discussion about personal responsibility and preferable waiting-room coffee brands.

5

And by the way, perhaps not the best time to bring it up . . . you all still owe me ten bucks.

If you had the patience to read this far, please show some support for my Aunt Teri, my new-found friend.

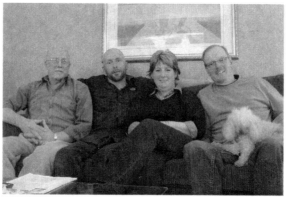

Michael's father, Michael, Auntie Teri, and Uncle Ray
Photo Courtesy of Teri Antcliffe

BE NOT MISTAKEN BY THE BELIEF
FRIDAY, APRIL 22, 2011 AT 11:26 PM

Let no one be mistaken by the belief that there is nothing one man nor woman can do against the enormous array of the worlds ills; against misery and ignorance, injustice and violence. Few of us will have the greatness to bend the course of history itself, but each of us can work and change a small portion of events. **In the sum total of these acts will be written the history of this generation!**

~ Robert F. Kennedy

WALL POST

You know you're dying the moment a doctor, who hasn't touched you without permission in three years, pats you on the knee.

FROM ANGELA
SATURDAY, APRIL 23, 2011 AT 3:23 PM

I would like to share *our* story with all of your current and new Facebook friends.

I am not surprised that Michael is doing this. I have always known him to put others first, even if his own life was in jeopardy. I know this first-hand because Michael saved my life back in elementary school.

We had all gone swimming one summer day at a neighbour's pond. I didn't know how to swim, so I floated around the pond on a rubber inner tube. One of our friends thought it would be a good idea to get on the same tube as me and then jump off. I moved over to let him on and, as soon as he jumped off, my tube flipped over. I was instantly in the water and was panicking because I didn't know how to swim. I was flailing around, coming up quickly, but more quickly sinking back down again. It was a sudden *fight for my life* situation.

All of our friends jumped in to help me, but I pushed them down and tried to stand on them in an attempt to get out of the water. They all struggled to help me, but my panic made me too strong. I remember sinking under the water and looking at the underside of the dock, floating on big oil drums. I remember seeing some oil leaking out, and thinking that some of the oil had been left in the drums. I also remember thinking *Oh my God. I am going to die.* I started to give up, but Michael didn't. He came back for probably his tenth fight with me and he finally managed to grab me and drag me out of the water. He pushed me up on top of the dock. We both lay there, completely exhausted. To this day I can't remember being as exhausted as I was then. We just lay there for a while and didn't say anything, just staring at each other. He had saved my life.

Michael never gave up. To this day, I am still terrified of water and I don't like to swim at all. When people ask me why, I tell them that I almost died from drowning once, but that my friend, Michael Antcliffe, saved my life. I miss you Michael. What you are doing is awesome. Keep strong and keep fighting. I wish I could save *your* life!

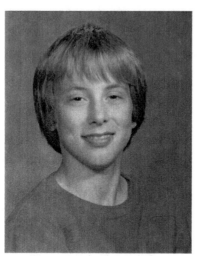

Young Michael Antcliffe

MY FAVOURITE CANCER MOMENTS THUS FAR . . . NO SPECIFIC ORDER
SATURDAY, APRIL 23, 2011 AT 7:28 PM

That day (three years ago) when we were pretty sure *we got it* with the second back excision was amazing. As I left the waiting room, I fought the urge to smile because I understood that there were more unfortunate souls sitting there. Clearly, I wasn't successful, because a woman saw me trying to hide my grin. This lady was the stereotypical cancer patient, complete with head-wrap. She gave me the biggest, most unashamed, most honest smile I have ever witnessed. This woman had walked a path with cancer that I had only touched on by this point. She had the strength to be happy for me. But, as much as I loved that moment, it wasn't until a couple of weeks ago that I realized I never saw her after that. Now that I'm one of those sitting in the waiting room I guess I'd better learn to smile . . .

Any time someone spends more than 30 seconds telling me how rough things are going for them was always an inside joke until now.

That reminds me of a cocky little 12-year-old I saw my first week of I.V. injections for immunotherapy, last September I think. It was starting to dawn on me that there was no one else my age around. All of these people were at least 15 to 20 years older than me, so I started mixing drinks for my pity party. Along came this head-wrap-wearing, grinning 12-year-old. This little bugger actually looked me up and down and I swear to god, as he passed, he popped his shoulders back at me as if to say, "Suck it up, buddy." And off he went . . . little shit. He did kinda remind me of someone, though.

The other day, an elderly lady offered a donation on behalf of her terminal husband. How do you say thank you for that and not learn your place in the grand scheme of things?

Nurse Karen is a great lady. She's been at all but one of my appointments, I think. She's honest and sincere, but with that *nothing fazes me* nurse-quality. She's awesome. She read my last test results, bit her lip a little, and then burst into tears. She gave me a big hug and excused herself. Her caring nature and the honesty of that moment will never leave my mind.

I've been staying with my friend, Pup, in Winnipeg for a week. We went to the Forks and I bought a rock with COURAGE engraved in it. I have kept it with me ever since. It reminds me of what I will need to hang onto to do this right. When I feel worried, I try to rub courage off the front; when I feel OK, I gently draw a circle with my finger on the smooth back side. We'll see which side lasts longer. I also settled on a cane that I feel best represents me. Every night at Pup's I have one in either hand. Had I left you all this week, my dear old friend Pup would have had to explain how he found me, "With his rock of courage in one hand and his pimp stick in the other!" He'll laugh out loud when he reads this.

You guys — the originals, and my new friends — are another memorable moment. I don't know what this process will give you, but I know it has already given me some peace and clarity. Talking to you, hearing your stories, and appreciating your efforts on my behalf have all taken an enormous weight off me. I suffer from fewer heavy breaths.

To you guys who know me, the nice things you've been saying don't make me seem half as full of myself as I did before.

Angela wrote and reminded me of the time I saved her from drowning, only a couple of weeks after I had learned to swim myself. Now she's married with a family of her own. Talk about a different perspective. One step left, one step right. A second too early, a second too late. This is what little control we have in our world. Time to start smelling the roses, people.

Call your mothers after reading this. Tell them they owe me ten bucks. Let's step through that little time portal that has become hope for me . . . back to a time where there was no such thing as a fight we weren't all in together.

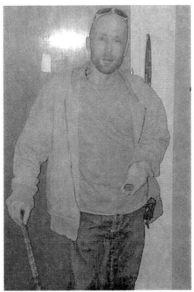

Michael, "with his rock of courage in one hand
and his pimp stick in the other"
Photo Courtesy of Seamus Collis

DEVOUT SINCERITY
SATURDAY, APRIL 23, 2011 AT 8:46 PM

In learning this path, it is only important to walk on the real ground, to act on the basis of reality. The slightest phoniness, and you fall into the realm of demons. If your vision is perfectly clear and you are not confused by objects twenty-four hours a day, then you gain power. If your vision does not penetrate freely, how can you do what is beyond measure?

~ **Liao-an**

That Liao-an fella, he comes over once a week and mows my lawn, then pays me a buck cause he's definitely giving me ten bucks in the end.

I love you guys. See you back in the Bay and convince your friends to care about you . . . and me too, please.

FROM ANNE

Michael Antcliffe and I met by chance when I was sent a link to his stunningly sensitive description of life with terminal cancer. Since then he has inspired me, heightened my perspective, and demonstrated a 360-degree view of courage on a daily basis.

Michael is fearless about sharing his experiences, especially his tests, treatments, and drug trials (with their inherent side effects) as he fights this seemingly unrelenting war. He has shared feelings about needing to win on a daily basis, when just getting through each day is a victory. This has struck a chord of recognition within my soul.

Not long ago, out of the blue, I found out that I had to have a biopsy. I didn't want to worry my family with how frightened I was. Late one night, I wrote to Michael and told him how I was feeling. True to form, he wrote right back, reassuring me and making the experience less terrifying. The results were negative and Michael was genuinely pleased for me.

If I had one wish (other than to take this scourge away) it would be that Michael could know just how much he has helped everyone with whom he is sharing this journey.

I am proud to call Michael my friend. His example continues to help me beyond measure. He has taught me how deeply you can care for someone that you have not met in-person. He has earned a special place in my heart where he will remain, regardless of what the future brings . . . ALWAYS.

WALL POST
SUNDAY, APRIL 24, 2011 AT 8:28 PM

My family has found the peace to cry openly. These days, every hug lingers a little longer. I needed this day to come so badly. I will lay my head down in true peace tonight. Thank you to all who have chosen to walk a few steps with me.

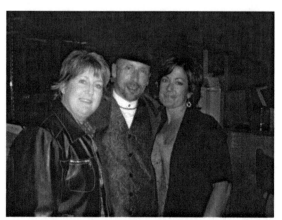

Auntie Teri, Michael and Michael's sister, Jennifer
Photo Courtesy of Teri Antcliffe

WHAT WE DO HERE . . .
WEDNESDAY, APRIL 27, 2011 AT 8:16 PM

I have really been struggling these past few days, trying to define a process that has become fluid before my eyes. I am in way over my head, but I have friends coming to my side. Clearly, I want to raise an impressive amount of cash for the care and comfort of those walking the last part of their paths with this disease. I want to provide as much peace and support as possible for people whose options have changed from preserving life to prolonging life. For me, this was the line that mattered most. But, if you look back to my first note, what I actually asked for was to have you walk a few steps with me and to volunteer to lose a friend . . . and to ask your friends to walk with you. My skepticism has taken a beating ever since. The sharing that people have done, the urgent desire to give, the words of support I have received – all of these things have been so much more than I expected. Initially my intent wasn't to go beyond local organizations or structures already in place, but to augment them. Now I don't want to leave out Turkey, Denmark, or Poland. Now I'm having language difficulties. This process is fluid; all of us can play a part in fine-tuning it. Let's put the money in a safe place (which for most of us is still the bank) and trust three of the best people I know to look over it. I haven't asked them yet because they will be putting themselves *out there* and it will be a lot of work, but worth it if my friends do their part and pay up at the end.

The charity name, if not taken, will be C-Cubed (power of three) Comfort Care for Cancer. I didn't get any suggestions for names, but do you guys like this one? What do you think of green font with the Sleeping Giant in the background? I'm open to suggestions . . .

For me, this is a release, a way of coping. This is my ego and me asking for the support of one million friends. This is my effort to provide a unique viewpoint to a question that gnaws at you. What the hell is wrong with this place? How do so many intelligent people, individuals, or groups do such stupid shit? How do we treat each other the way we do and not suffer from shame? How do we not know our neighbours' first and last names? How did we come to invent the term *bystander apathy* and not do anything about it? How will we reach our goals? How will we know when and where that moment happens? How did we get suckered into listening to this self-righteous little shit? Permit me this, please, my friends. I feel as though my pace has quickened these past seven months. I feel as though I have broken from the pack, rushed ahead foolishly, and I now find myself looking back. I'm seeing things with an entirely new perspective. I'm seeing these friends gather around: from childhood, from school, from work, and kids I've helped care for. It is not by accident that we found each other in this community and I want to visit with as many of you as possible. Those who brought us to the mighty 1,000, we'll get to know one another. And how about my re-friending of Aunt Teri! It won't take another decade for us to break bread.

You other guys — keep being honest with me. Tell me when I'm a pompous ass. Make jokes, laugh, and cry with me. Open your minds to the possibility that I may have unique insight. After all, I'm the only one who figured a way out of this without paying ten bucks. Muhahahahahahah!

A FLUID PROCESS
SATURDAY, APRIL 30, 2011 AT 3:38 PM

Facebook is a crazy thing to begin to understand. The mutual friend icon is revealing many things (don't worry, I'm pretty sure stars compress before they explode). Motivating the people right beside you is often very hard. I'll be honest . . . looking over my original list, I hoped I would have spoken to almost all of my friends by now since my ability to remember names is so much better for some reason. On the bus trip I took to Winnipeg, Bruce (a young cook heading to Calgary) sat beside me. I'll likely never see him again, but I won't forget his name. Stephan (a German kid doing a working tour of North America) rode with me on the way back. I love the fact that people are calling out their friends to explain their inaction. I had hoped at the outset of this to do something together, for us to speak and act in unison, and thus reaffirm the fact that our meaningful interaction can draw a million people closer together. Little interconnected groups of groups of people left to speak as one. Imagine any issue or cause needing support, and imagine saying, "Let's put a million people on that problem today!"

But here, we cannot afford apathy or inaction. We cannot go softly into the dark night. We must step firmly and leave our footprints behind so our friends may follow. We cannot seek excuses for the time we were not given or the breaks we didn't get. Here, we cannot afford the time necessary to shake our fists at the gods. To get to 1,000,000, to raise such funds for people in need, we must live lives of meaning and not single-serving convenience. And we

19

must approach our friends in the same regard.

We cannot afford phrases like, "Oh well, what can you do . . . That's the way it is . . . I'm only one person." Apathy is its own cancer, especially among good friends, so let's not be afraid to question one another and speak openly. Let's look at the taken-for-granted nature of our world and question each bit of it! If we do not speak openly and frankly with one another, we cannot name our fears. If we cannot name our fears, we cannot take power from them and defeat them.

We can remove fear through language and laughter. Think of how fast the *C-word* can shut up an entire room (or a Greyhound bus from Winnipeg). This isn't the *C-word* from my youth. That was another word you were never supposed to use because it was vulgar and disrespectful. We can take back the *C-word* and make it something else. Let's just mess over some other word that can be the new Voldemort *He-Who-Must-Not-Be-Named* (Harry Potter reference). When we don't speak openly, we're just putting on blinders. I just did it for three years, at each stage putting off consideration of the next. Everyone around you knows it's there, just not what to say or ask. It makes me feel like I'm six and my parents are spelling things out in front of me to shield me from some reality so I don't freak out about the existence of c-o-o-k-i-e-s (not a candidate for the new *C-word*).

My active cancer, all these damned mystery lumps, my pain . . . I need them to have a name and I need them to be real for you and me. In a world of superficial platitudes and catch-phrase communication, it is still possible to connect meaningfully with one another and to take power from something as imposing as cancer, not to mention the other things about this world that we fear but do not speak of.

I can't stop what I've started. I can't click my heels together and wish cancer away anymore, pretending my path is the yellow brick road. I can't change the way I walk this path either, though: the concept of living one's life backwards is too entrenched in my mind. My love for Mother Earth has taught me too much humility to reach elsewhere for answers at this point in life. Samurai were said to have lived life backwards. Once one has embraced the inevitability of his own departure from this world, then true personal responsibility and active social conscience are possible. One becomes able to speak with devout sincerity. After the who, the what, the where, the when and the why are established, we still decide the how. On this path together, when members of our tribe fall, we will pay homage to the how — how they fought and died and how they chose to live their lives.

And here we will, as friends, discover the true measure of one whispering voice caught amid the roar of a million who follow. Here we will be humble, but not meek. We can exclude no one from participating because cancer doesn't see the imaginary lines we draw to make sense of this world. When death comes knocking on my door, I'm gonna introduce him to a million good friends. I'm going to have to ask him about that ten bucks I lent him so many years ago.

CONNECTIONS . . .
SUNDAY, MAY 8, 2011 AT 11:30 AM

Talk about making connections . . . Diane, head of the Daylin James fan club (world-famous local-talent Elvis impersonator) has offered me two tickets to tonight's show at the Auditorium. Diane called Fran, whose sons I went to school with. Fran called my father, and my father called me. That's pretty ninja. Look for my mother and me at tonight's show. Thank you Diane, Fran, and Daylin James. Oh, and all 2,425 of you guys.

WALL POST
SUNDAY, MAY 8, 2011 AT 11:39 PM

Elvis (Daylin James) was awesome. He did even better as his own opening act. Go to see him sing if you get the chance. Thanks to the work of his fan club (thank you ladies), Elvis announced my birthday and Facebook mission to the crowd. Very cool connection.

MY CANCER . . .
SUNDAY, MAY 8, 2011 AT 2:14 PM

It's been on my mind for the past week or so to just write something about cancer. The more I struggle to think of something profound or eye opening, the more I realize that I'm wholly unqualified. Talking with many of you these past few weeks has shown me this. I can't tell you what it's like to have cancer. After having so many people share their stories and life situations with me, it has become very clear to me that I know very little about cancer in general, but I do know *my cancer*, and I am beginning to understand why cancer patients own it and call it *my cancer*. Other people don't ask how your fight with cancer is going. They use phrases like, "how's cancer?" or, "how's the cancer thing going?" I even recall once being asked, "how's your cancer doing?" Strange priorities are revealed in *that* question. Well . . . *my cancer* is doing just fine, unfortunately, but I thought I'd take the time to say exactly how fine.

In May of 2008, I had a birthmark removed from between my shoulder blades along with a subsequent excision to ensure that no cancer remained. I had suffered an injury to that part of my body years earlier, but it wasn't until a friend suggested I get it checked that I realized a part of it had grown back all on its own. Two minor excisions later, my odds were still pretty good, but I appreciated the fact that years had already passed. I found out that I first had cancer while standing in line at Tim Hortons (whole other story). I recall doing a flooring job for a woman who had a variety of medical issues, including cancer. When my boss

23

commented that I was also a cancer survivor of melanoma, her response was, "Oh no, I had *real* cancer."

In late June 2010, a lymph node in my left armpit began to swell. It grew for a few weeks and then just maintained itself . . . sort of. In August, I had a *radical auxiliary dissection* of ten left-side lymph nodes. Whoever wrote the report described the largest node as "huge" (7 cm by 4.5 cm by 4 cm). Under microscopic examination, "the largest node is completely replaced by an extensively necrotic melanin producing metastatic malignant melanoma." It was a little cancer factory, in other words. Aside from recovering from surgery, life didn't change too much around me. But I had done the homework and I knew I had a 10% chance of making it five years from diagnosis. For me, life still didn't change that much. I healed; I started a year-long cycle of immunotherapy; I went back to work. My doctor continued to scan me to see if the drugs were keeping cancer away.

This stage of cancer also introduced me to the two mystery lumps discovered in my left lung, four in my liver, and others in the subcutaneous tissue of my left abdomen. More have since developed and, although two can be felt from the outside, none can be seen.

This past April, the results from a CT scan showed abnormalities in my spine. Subsequent PET and MRI scans showed that cancer had returned in my bones in at least three different spots. A "destructive lesion" on my L3 vertebrae, right scapula and pelvic bone has appeared. A tiny T7 metastasis cannot be excluded from the count. Had cancer only come back into my spine, an operation may have stopped it. I kinda want to find that lady and ask her if *my cancer* is real enough now.

I'm as guilty as the next guy (or that lady) for first treating *my cancer* like a sissy version of the disease. It wasn't until I heard that it couldn't be stopped that I began to pay it the respect it deserves. When the technician refers to you in a report as, ". . . an unfortunate patient with melanoma," it's time to take the blinders off. My vision has never been clearer. I don't have sissy cancer; I have bloody ninja cancer. *My cancer,* apparently, reads up on its Sun Tzu and has studied the battlefield. *My cancer* hit me where I would have in its position — my strong arm and my back. None of this truly hurt until four months ago. After the chemo was stopped, because it wasn't really working, I realized that my pain is not chemo pain, it's actually *my cancer.* So I only really know why *my cancer* sucks, and I've only truly appreciated this just recently.

My cancer sucks because I've only seen it twice, and it's only taken three swings at me. It sucks that I've never had an opportunity to swing back . . . until now. *My cancer* sucks because you really can't see it in me when I pass you on the street. *My cancer* hasn't taken me off my feet yet, but it's spreading in that direction. *My cancer* has slowly removed my strength and endurance. I need to lay down twice a day to relieve the pressure on my spine. The day my body told me I needed a cane, I went out and bought one. I lean on things constantly. My gas tank quickly empties during the day and doesn't refill itself completely anymore. Now, with the help of painkillers, I understand the curative effects of Metamucil. I'm 35 years-old. *My cancer* sucks because when it came back into my lymph nodes, I also went deaf in my left ear, which now only registers a loud, constant, high-pitched ringing. The ringing has now started in my right ear. No doctor has told me that the two are related, but cancer is the only scapegoat I have for now.

The worst part is that no one can really tell, but I can, and I know that cancer has yet to begin to truly take from me. Four months ago, I could carry two bundles of shingles up a two-story ladder. I could muscle a 4′x8′ sheet of decking around like nothing. I could walk all day long. Now I take every opportunity to rest and conserve energy; now my pimp stick feels more comfortable every day. There is a certain peace to be found in having choice removed from oneself, from realizing that nothing is truly in your hands. But this path is short, and I must make use of every moment. *My cancer* now gets to see me dig my heels in and go a little ninja myself. I have a plan for *my cancer*, and it doesn't involve dying quite yet. When cancer does take that last swing at me, it better have ten bucks in its other hand. On this ride we all pay the boatman.

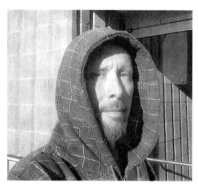

Michael is ready to go ninja

WALL POST
FRIDAY, MAY 13, 2011 AT 7:50 AM

I thought that having a CAT scan first thing on the morning of my birthday would suck. Having hundreds of well-wishes to wake up to really takes the suckiness away. You guys are awesome. Today, people, we slay dragons all day long, no matter how big and tough they think they are. Love you guys.

WALL POST
SUNDAY, MAY 15, 2011 AT 10:00 PM

The plan is to suck up the next three weeks of chemo/radiation, while planning the specifics of my East Coast road trip. I have the car and the travelling companion, but not the exact destinations (minus capital cities). I need to find the best fishing spots on the way and the cool attractions.

WALL POST
Tuesday, May 17, 2011 at 7:20 AM

I'm disappointed. It has been more than 12 hours since radiation treatment and still no evidence of emerging superpowers. I asked that the machine be set somewhere between Spider-Man and the Incredible Hulk. Maybe it's the chemo. I'll ask them to turn up the juice today. If I'm a pain in the butt now, just wait until I'm big, green, and angry.

WALL POST
Wednesday, May 18, 2011 at 9:40 AM

Good morning campers. I have three days left of treatment and three days left until fishing. Have fun today. If you use an elevator at any point, once the doors close, face the back of the elevator instead of staring like sheep at the floor numbers, and then start a conversation with the first person to make eye contact. It'll mess them up for the rest of the day. Then tell them they owe me ten bucks.

SUPERPOWERS
WEDNESDAY, MAY 18, 2011 AT 5:09 PM

I'm sure someone had their fingers crossed, because I'm quite certain I found my superpowers today. It turns out they work for the Thunder Bay Regional Health Sciences Foundation and the Northern Cancer Research Fund. The wealth of knowledge and experience found there, along with the help of a website called Canada Helps (gotta love the name), I believe puts all the necessary ducks in a row. I find high spirits even further renewed today. Distant goals seem not so far off. Mine is one million people walking the same path. I was once told that a man's reach should far exceed his grasp. You and I, my friends, shall reach far and wide. We will have our voices heard and our footprints followed.

GLITCH IN THE PLAN
Tuesday, May 24, 2011 at 10:01 PM

The original plan . . .

   While working as a youth care worker, I contributed to an RPP (Registered Pension Plan) that I could cash in through a shortened life expectancy clause. I just have to pay the taxes and get roughly $6,000.00–$7,000.00. The plan: buy a laptop and an iPhone, head to the East Coast with my old man, meet as many of you crazy people on the way as I can, and fish every second stream or lake . . . and hopefully raise a bunch of cash for cancer. I completely underestimated the complexity of setting up a charity fund and getting an iPhone. My superpowers helped (Thunder Bay Regional Health Science Centre and Northern Cancer Research Fund) take most of my worries away. The RPP should be in my bank account soon. I already have my new laptop and most of my route is planned. I've even found the least-expensive (still pretty expensive) deal I could on renting a car for a month, but I'm sure it'll be more comfy on my bones than my dad's no-suspension truck.

I've been busy these last few weeks arranging to move in with my father, arranging my own finances through EI and CPP disability, fishing over May long weekend, and trying to meet friends (both old and new). I feel like I've somewhat neglected you guys.

At the beginning of next month I get a press conference. I get an easy, secure way for people to donate money (Google "Canada Helps") and help in understanding social media a lot more. My father will have moved in with me, and my financing will be arranged (fingers crossed).

The earliest I can leave now is the 11th or 12th of next month. Last week I decided to do a week of radiation treatment, as well as chemotherapy (dacarbazine). I need to do at least two rounds of the chemo to see if it is having any effect, and the next round ends on the 10th of June. Then I'm on the road (come hell or high water) so anyone who lives east of Thunder Bay can look out for me. Destinations so far include Brampton, Toronto (Zoo), Ottawa, Montreal, Quebec City, and (Camp) Petawawa. I know PEI and Nova Scotia are in, but I don't know if Newfoundland is possible. I have everything I need except communication on the road, so I'll have to rely on Wi-Fi and the laptop. Anyone with plan suggestions?

A POEM FROM ONE OF MY NEW
FRIENDS . . .
WEDNESDAY, MAY 25, 2011 AT 6:26 PM

Shhh . . . It's gone now
Don't make a sound
I know it's hovering very near
But I'm afraid to look around
I'll hide here where it's quiet
As only painlessness can be
And I cannot help but wonder
If it will ever set me free

The enemy is senseless and sadistic
I'm at the mercy of its every whim
And in my darkest hours
I'm certain I'll never be free of him

Suddenly searing rockets of pain
Illuminate my hiding place
And I know he's lurking right nearby
Though I cannot see his face

As I struggle to arm myself
For this newest battle just begun
I know he'll never be the victor
Until I acknowledge that he's won

Strengthened by this brief respite
I head into the fray
Knowing I'll do my level best
To survive even one more day

I smile when I realize I don't know his strength
Or does he mine
It may be over in a minute
But at this SECOND I'm just fine

~ **Anne Raynor, 1985**

A MORNING FILLED WITH PERSPECTIVE . . .
SATURDAY, JUNE 4, 2011 AT 11:01 AM

It's 9:31 AM my time, and it's been a hell of a day already. I woke up at 5:30 in pain, so my day began with the realization that my current regimen of painkillers isn't working. I'm not using very powerful painkillers, but each increase in dosage is a litmus test for how I'm doing, just like the stairs at the Cancer Centre are a litmus test for still having my feet underneath me. I bought a brace yesterday with lumbar support and it works great. I put it in the same category as the pimp stick. Both are items I still feel I don't absolutely need; however, both are items my body is thankful for from the moment I began using them. It's tough for a guy like me to have a battle going on between pride and logic. Both run strong inside of me. My perspective on how I view myself is changing, just as the perspective of others changes when they see me with my cane.

As I was returning from getting coffee this morning, two dogs poked their noses in the gate of my apartment building. Most people wouldn't call two strange dogs into their yard, but I strongly advocate petting strange dogs. Had I not called them in, they may have wandered onto the adjoining train tracks or four-lane street. So I posted pics of two very nice, very tired and wet, strange dogs that had clearly been chasing skunks recently. It made me quite happy that I could help return them to their owner. While waiting for the owner to arrive, my friend Shawn texted me to tell me that a mutual friend had lost her seven-year-old today to cancer. I don't

34

include her name out of respect, but trust me, if you knew her life you would understand why I hope that I have her strength. The owner arrived to see me in tears, but was still quite happy about finding her dogs. I can only imagine her perspective on the day.

On my way back from my second cup of coffee, I stopped to talk to a guy I see and say good morning to every day. The first real conversation with him began with him asking me why I'm limping. I told him it's due to cancer. He immediately told me of a friend in the hospital who had lost both legs and, soon after, one of his arms in his fight against cancer. All were amputated in an effort to preserve his life. This man can't bear to visit his friend any longer. It immediately made me consider both his, and especially his friend's, perspective on life today.

I then made the mistake of watching the news. It saddened me to learn that Terry Fox's mom is very ill. I went to her son's memorial just the other day. This woman and her family have gone more than the whole nine yards in fighting cancer. They gave all that they had and more. The streaming text at the bottom of the screen then revealed yet another soulless prick using cancer to steal money (and from Canadian veterans at that). Talk about resetting the bar for selfish bastards everywhere. Two stories, side-by-side: one about national concern and loss, the other about soon-to-be national shame. Some folks behave like angels, while some folks fall to the path of demons. It depends on whether or not we live according to our own perspective, and whether or not we try, every now and then, to see things from one another's perspective.

Then a local rock radio host, Mark Tannahill, commented on one of my posts, which got me thinking that he and I (along with the fine people of Marsville and Kakabeka) all share at least one similar perspective.

Then, fishing got cancelled. Any other day this would have pissed me off, but with all things in perspective, it's not that big a deal.

Now my brain kinda hurts and I'm trying to put this whole morning and my entire Facebook adventure into perspective. The other day, a woman posted a question about why someone would accept a friend request from someone they didn't know. It was a harmless and valid question from her perspective. She only asked because the friend who suggested this to her didn't fully explain why she should befriend me, I imagine. Some of us kinda snapped at this innocent lady (from our own perspective of course). I appreciate that some of you are quite defensive of me, but I believe those of us here now need to act like elders to those new followers to come. We will be the ones who explain and clarify our purpose here, the ones who share with each other, the ones who create and appreciate each connection made with a new friend. We need to be the ones who welcome all with open arms, because cancer touches everyone without taking any perspective at all.

I've been asked, "Do I know you?" very often, so here's the perspective I think we should take for the day, all 3,483 of us. My press release got delayed 'til the 9th, which gives us five days until the fan page opens up. Let's not get impatient with the number of people; they will come. Let's worry about *us* for now, the same *us* that is saturated with mutual friends who have begun finding their own connections as part of this. Only half of us need to get one more person to become my Facebook friend for this page to reach 5,000 within the next five days. Then, once the page is active and advertised, this 5,000 can set the bar for those to come. This group puts the first footsteps down so that others can follow. There's no point in making the next friend you find an easy task. I am going after the only friend I ever took off my Facebook list, a woman who was once my best friend and that I haven't spoken to in two years — a woman whose son I loved as though he were my own. The issue that came between us seems smaller each day. I encourage you all to do the same.

Find a family member you've been quarreling with, find a friend you haven't spoken to in years, or find someone you have issues with. Hell, find someone you know who hates your guts, because it doesn't matter what you're fighting about, what the issues are, or where the hate came from . . . it's all a matter of perspective. And as time draws short, perspectives have a tendency to change. Let logic win over pride today. Be someone who finds a tough-to-find friend today, tell them you're happy you found them, and tell them they should owe me ten bucks. Remember how history spoke of 300 brave Spartans? Imagine the story of 3,483 . . .

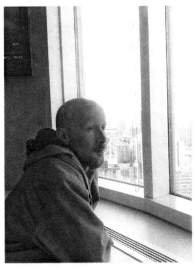

Looking for perspective
Photo Courtesy of Hayley McLeod

WALKING IN THE LIGHT . . .
TUESDAY, JUNE 7, 2011 AT 9:45 AM

The mutual objective recognition of minds was called transmission of the lamp. Perfectly clear spiritual knowledge taught in accord with potentials. There were some, however, who sunk into voidness and lingered in stillness . . . not knowing for themselves that the body is the site of enlightenment. Their every thought was on objects, turning away from awakening. Retreating and forgetting halfway along the path, they sank forever into the realm of devils.

~ **P'uan**

FROM KATHY
(IN AN EMAIL TO MICHAEL)

I have a story.

Today while at work . . . ok . . . wait, back up . . . I look after a guy that is palliative and has been for a while. Anyway, he was a really, *really* bad dude before he ended up with a brain injury. He can't talk now, but he can parrot what other people say. He has been bedridden for over a year, with no TV, stimulation, or family. It's really very sad.

Back to today . . . while I was feeding him his supper, I thought of you, and I looked at this man and thought that he needed to smile. So I started to sing, "You better watch out, you better not cry. . ." and he started singing too. That was fun, so then I thought maybe he would like to *see* some singing. Again, I was thinking of you. So, given his age and history, I got out my iPhone and decided to find him a song. I don't know why, but the song "The Wreck of the Edmund Fitzgerald" by Gordon Lightfoot came to mind. So I typed it in and, like a child seeing television for the very first time, he watched it. His lips curled up and he smiled. And then (I thought he was getting tired) he was wiping tears.

Now I have looked after this man for many years. He is not very responsive on his own, but he looked at me after we watched the video and said, "Thank you." As I left him I was grinning from ear-to-ear and I said to myself, *Damn that Michael Antcliffe!*

I have learned to spend a few extra minutes with my patients, because I don't know how long they have or how long *I* have for that matter, and *every* extra moment counts! So, I thought I'd say thanks. And, since I work this weekend, I am bringing in my notebook computer and I am gonna sit with that man and pull up some good tunes and let him watch and smile.

I just had to share this with you, to show you that everything you are teaching us and talking about and sharing really, *really* does matter! I am an old dog learning new tricks.

WALL POST
SUNDAY, JUNE 12, 2011 AT 9:37 AM

It's gonna be hot today . . . sunscreen people! I really can't emphasize this enough. Wait . . . yes I can.

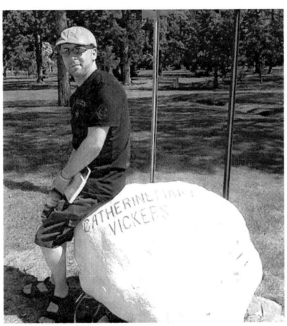

Michael visiting Vicker's Park (Thunder Bay, ON)

MY BUDDY PETE . . .
TUESDAY, JUNE 14, 2011 AT 12:33 PM

I've been meaning to tell you more about my buddy Pete. If there's one thing that could sum Pete up, it's the stolen sign at the end of his driveway, which reads *Redneck Blvd.* Pete has spent more time hunting and fishing than most people spend working. He has subsisted off of more wild game than any other man I know. Pete doesn't trust the government, police, lawyers, doctors, or pretty much anyone with more than a Grade 12 education. Every word that comes out of Pete's mouth is completely unfiltered. Situational appropriateness and political correctness don't always register with him. Everything he says is delivered with the same candor and passion. Pete can lie to you about the size of fish he caught and bluff shamelessly in poker, but there is no real falsehood or deception in the man. If the show "Survivor" was real, Pete would win it all and call everyone who finished after him a pussy. When Pete first saw me, after we learned that cancer had made it to my bones, he looked me dead in the eye and without any expression on his face, clearly stated, "It gets worse." That, in a morbid nutshell, is why you just gotta love Pete. Even when societal norms dictate some degree of watering down of the truth or kind pleasantries, Pete comes out in unaltered high-definition every time.

I put Pete right in the middle of the grey area that is 99% of humanity. A changing mixture of good and bad, he never strays too far to either extreme. We're all just a collection of attitudes learned through life experiences, combined with the culturally-learned behaviour we individually become accepting of and comfortable with. There are few purely good or evil people in the world, but those are just the ones who make the news on a daily basis. Finding someone to tell you the unwavering truth (painful or otherwise) is becoming more and more rare with each passing day. We spend so much time discussing matters of trivial importance and being fearful of the unknown that we deprive ourselves of the natural richness and depth of human interaction. We communicate with one another in a single-serving manner, using tools that encourage ease and expediency over real and meaningful interaction. There's nothing quite like the spoken truth to cut through the cloud of confusion. Pete understands this, though you couldn't convince him to care.

I spent the first two years of my fight with cancer never questioning or contemplating any of the things people said to me. I would just listen blankly as all the automatic and expected phrases were uttered. People touted the wonders of modern medicine and fantastic cures that just never quite made it to market. People would explain the odds of this and that, leaving me wondering why, for the first time in my life, everyone is telling me how good I look, and so on. It's nice to hear, but the truth is that people tell you how good you look because you don't fit the image of someone who's dying from cancer. They're commenting on how good you look . . . so far. The truth is that advice about keeping up hope rarely comes with directions about where to find it. The same people who told me not to worry and to stay positive are the same ones who very smoothly transitioned into telling me I could have more time than the percentages suggest. The truth is that these automatic phrases are spoken so easily because we're all afraid, and we all become more uncomfortable and fearful when the need to confront our fears becomes unavoidable.

Cancer is no different from a schoolyard bully who survives on intimidation and fear. My father's advice to me as a child regarding fighting was, "If someone pushes you, swing first. You are already in a fight; you just need to decide the stakes." You don't have to beat the bully senseless, so long as he learns that each time he comes to impose his will, you're ready to fight tooth and nail. It's the same kind of logic that led me to grow a seven-month playoff beard during the first round of chemo as a daily reminder (whenever I looked in the mirror), like a little eff you to cancer. I think what I'm really hoping to do here is to call out the bully, speak openly and without fear, have some laughs and good times at its expense and, by doing so, take the power of fear and intimidation from it.

There's nothing like bouncing an idea off a few thousand people in order to define and enrich a concept like hope. It's definitely one thing we have yet to put in environmentally destructive, yet oh so convenient, six-packs. But once you learn to spot it or accept its presence amid a sea of doubt, it starts to find you everywhere. You can only hear so many stories about strength in the face of adversity, or celebration in spite of loss, before you naturally begin to pick out your own little moments of hope. It's like having moments stored away for when your mettle is truly tested. I find these moments everywhere these days: in your efforts made on my behalf, stories and questions from friends (old and new), people telling me they are connecting more closely with one another and treating time with the respect it deserves. I see hope in the sweet elderly women in the yellow volunteer shirts at the chemo clinic. I'm sure each of them could take me to school when it comes to loss and hope, so I hope we can all continue to call out the bully. Hope is often found in places where you least expect it. I want this place to be where people come and ask for directions, so long as my buddy Pete isn't doing his community service at the front desk.

Pete didn't find out about his colon cancer until well into the fourth stage. The first option given to him was basically no option at all. None, at least, that the mind is prepared for until a drastic change in perspective occurs. So, he spared no expense in promptly going to the far side of the planet, killing some of Mother Earth's finest creatures and placing their conquered heads on his wall. Pete went and purchased a 25-foot cabin cruiser and is spending the summer touring the Trent-Severn Waterway. I may not see Pete again, but I'm confident that he's spending each day doing what matters most to him. I'm also confident that he's giving his own little eff you to cancer each day.

Pete was predictably upfront about telling me there was no damn way I was getting ten bucks out of him.

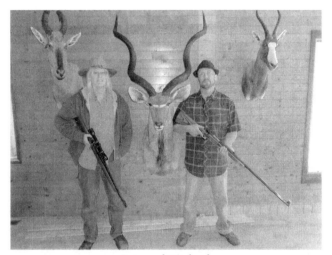

Pete and Michael

WALL POST
Tuesday, June 14, 2011 at 1:04 PM

Today fishing (original, I know) is my little eff you to cancer. I encourage everyone to find their own, or just go fishing. See you later.

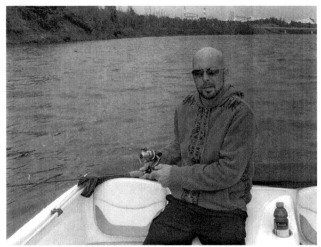

Michael fishing
Photo Courtesy of Mike Robbins

WALL POST
THURSDAY, JUNE 16, 2011 AT 12:08 PM

Fishing cancelled on account of a broken canoe yesterday. Today I visit a friend in the hospital and tomorrow . . . something else will probably come up. We need to organize a big group fishing trip . . . or derby, yaaaaaaaaaaa. See you soon.

WALL POST
THURSDAY, JUNE 16, 2011 AT 8:34 PM

Today has been a draining day, early to bed tonight. Sleep well — the early bird gets the worm . . . thus, the worm that sleeps in gets to live another day.

TOO FUNNY...
SATURDAY, JUNE 18, 2011 AT 8:14 PM

Thanks to Jolene (whose Facebook post I stole this from).

BREAKING NEWS: The Pity Train has just derailed at the intersection of Suck It Up & Move On, and crashed into We All Have Problems, before coming to a complete stop at Get the Heck Over It. Any complaints about how we operate can be forwarded to 1-800-WAA-WAAA. This is Dr. Sniffle Reporting LIVE from Quitchur Fussin'. If you like this, repost it. If you don't . . . suck it up cupcake! Life doesn't revolve around you.

FROM CHRISTINE

I became Facebook friends with Michael Antcliffe in April of 2011 when one of my friends suggested that I add him as a friend. I met him for the first time in person when he did his press conference at the Thunder Bay Regional Health Sciences Centre. I've seen him at the hospital many times since then when he attends various appointments at the Cancer Centre. I have had the pleasure of being able to meet with him for coffee when he has the time. I'm not sure how long it was after meeting him on Facebook that I decided to visit his page every morning and leave him a *Good Morning* message. I hoped that I could bring a smile to his face and help get his day off to a good start. I've continued to do so every day, with only a few days missed because of various circumstances.

I'm so glad that I chose to become Michael's friend and embark on this journey with him. It has made me look at life from a different perspective, and not take so many things for granted. He inspires me with the way he faces his disease head-on. He never falters, no matter what obstacles he is faced with. I have diabetes and I know that when I was in my teens and twenties I was always thinking to myself, *why me?*, not realizing how lucky I was to have a disease that could be controlled, as long as I took the initiative to take care of myself. However, Michael doesn't have the same options that I do in being able to control his disease, and yet he still fights his battle in a positive way, never letting it conquer him. By joining him on his journey, I have made the conscious decision to think more about others and to stand by people who don't have the opportunities that I have. There are many struggles that others face every day, without any options available to them to help make their lives easier.

Because of all I have learned from Michael while joining him on his journey, I had the idea of getting a team together, with Michael, for the Relay for Life this year. I'm very grateful that he was honoured by the idea and has become our team captain. By doing this, I feel I am able to do something for him to thank him for all that he has taught me about this horrible disease and the many things that are involved in fighting a battle against it. I have also learned quite a bit about malignant melanoma and agree that we need to get the information out about this disease, especially to the younger generation, so that people know about the increased possibility of developing melanoma if they are not careful.

So, in closing, I would like to thank Michael for allowing me to join him on his journey against malignant melanoma and say that I am glad to be one of his supporters. If you haven't joined him in his battle, please do so. You will see what I am talking about. I look forward to the Relay for Life in June and helping him raise money to destroy this horrible disease.

THINGS I'VE LEARNED TO APPRECIATE THUS FAR . . . NO SPECIFIC ORDER
THURSDAY, JUNE 23, 2011 AT 6:54 PM

I appreciate my oncologist because he has the exact qualities I expect a doctor to have and he looks and acts like I expect a doctor to. I don't know how important that really is, but at the very least it's reassuring. I appreciate that he likes to use complicated medical jargon as much as I like to listen to it, but I've never once felt like he was insulting my intelligence. I appreciate that he only takes 15 minutes to actually describe any test results or change in treatment, but still takes another 15 minutes to answer any questions I ask. I appreciate that he speaks softly, but that each word carries the same level of confidence. I do my homework when it comes to my condition and my options. I appreciate the fact that I've only ever stumped him with one question, and he was wise enough to answer that it was in God's hands. I appreciate that more than once I've seen him working under a desk lamp at the nurse's station, long after clinic hours were over and everyone else had left. I appreciate that I'm saying all of this despite the fact that the man's good news/bad news ratio with me is less than stellar. I appreciate that it's someone's job to find things in his office from time to time. I appreciate that few will actually get that reference, but trust me, the people who do are having a good snicker.

I appreciate my surgeon and my radiation doctor for the same reasons. They both did exactly what they said they could and would do. They both exude the same confidence that would lead you to throw them the keys when faced with the need for a high

51

speed chase.

There's a host of other people involved in making the Cancer Centre run the way it does. Many I can see and many are behind the scenes. I spent the first part of this fight trying to forget them and everything else about that place. Now I appreciate each of them, what they deal with daily, and the strength it takes to do such things daily. Now there is no place I would rather be cared for.

I appreciate the people I met from a company called Elekta, and their friend, Karen. They played a pivotal role in bringing our efforts here into the light and they are some truly genuine people. They took one small step out of their way to lend a hand and expected nothing in return, which is rare these days.

I appreciate people who deal with chronic pain. I now appreciate that pain can eat away at you, not simply through its severity, but also through its unceasing nature. Thus, I now have new appreciation for each physical step I take on this path, from the first painful one in the morning to the last peaceful one at night.

I appreciate the elderly and the infirm, mostly because on a bad day some of you are now passing me on the stairs. Honestly, I've become impatient waiting for some of you in the past. Now you can get in my way all day long, take as long as you like to decide what kind of Danish you want while I wait behind you in line, and you can tell me how it was in the old days. I've got time for that now. Just as motorcyclists and Jeep drivers always wave to one another, so too should those of use with canes, walkers or wheelchairs.

I appreciate the mercy I've found in the fact that I will never have to watch a member of my immediate family go through this.

I appreciate the peace I've found in this journey. At this point in my life, there are no wrongs I still need to right and no apologies I must make before I go. I appreciate the manner in which I've walked my path. I do not need to change now.

I appreciate that people greet me with hugs far more often than before and they always tell me how good I look. I don't understand why we wait until people are dying to do this. I believe we should institute both as a common greeting.

I appreciate some of the simplest things I do. People I see and places I go are part of a bucket list. I appreciate each of these people, places, and things so much more richly and deeply because of this, which is another thing I wish I'd have learned to do years ago.

I appreciate the fact that the greater our numbers grow, the greater is the likelihood that I may not be the first member of this tribe to fall. Mine is not the only tale of woe to be found among us.

I appreciate the comfort in finding the only person I've ever deleted from Facebook. She's added another beautiful kid and a hubby to her family. It's a step I always told her she needed to take. I appreciate that our reconnection felt like old times, as opposed to mumbling curse words under my breath at her.

And, not least of all, I appreciate you guys. I appreciate each word of kindness or encouragement, each question, each response, and each story you've shared. I appreciate the continued efforts of all of you, and I appreciate the patience and ingenuity we must have to stay this course. I appreciate that it isn't always easy to convince someone to owe a total stranger ten bucks, and then convince them to go out and convince someone else to do the same. I appreciate the hell out of the fact that so many of you continue to do so.

ONE DAY DELAY
Wednesday, July 6, 2011 at 11:38 AM

Our trip is delayed until early tomorrow. I'm off to load up the laptop with movies and music. I saw the specialist this morning about the deafness/ringing in my left ear, which is so much better than the witch doctor I saw last time about it. It turns out a $4,000.00 hearing aid-type device connected to a screw implanted in my skull would help quite a bit . . . so, unfortunately, the deafness and ringing will have to be tolerated. I'm not prepared to go all Borg (Star Trek reference) at this point in life. The ringing can't be fixed either way. I'll be back later, but tomorrow at this time I will be headed for Pancake Bay for the first night of the road trip. I'll post my itinerary in a note later tonight. Have a good day guys.

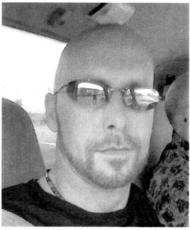

Michael on his way to the East Coast

THE RESULTS OF OUR EFFORTS . . .
FRIDAY, JULY 8, 2011 AT 12:55 PM

It's bright and early on Day Two of the road trip. We're travelling down the Trans-Canada in the mighty Ford Ranger. Thus far, the trip has been pretty cool. I've seen some neat beaches and coves, and soaked up a lot of beautiful landscapes while travelling east. We've just left the Soo and are now heading for Southern Ontario. Unfortunately, the day before we left, I accidentally broke my pimp stick in the car door. I've found a cheap replacement for the time being, but finding a permanent new one is a side mission for this trip.

As you may have noticed, Tracie Smith posted that almost $4,000.00 has been raised for the care of people with cancer thus far. I don't believe that this includes anonymous donations or ones dropped off at the Northern Cancer Fund office. Regardless, it's a measure of what we have achieved thus far. Clearly this figure doesn't match with 3,850 people giving ten bucks apiece, but you can look at it in many different ways. It works out to almost $500.00 per week since this began, or a 10% response rate from Facebook friends, or simply $4,000.00 that wasn't available for cancer patients before we started. I prefer to look at it as the equivalent of 400 people promising to do something and then following through with it. For a total stranger, the satisfaction of helping a fellow human being is their only reward. I'd like to thank the people who gave what they said they would, as well as those who went above and beyond with their generosity. I much prefer to look to the 10% accumulated so far rather than the 90% that's yet to come. If you don't share my point of view, then my advice to you is to avoid cancer at all costs and wear your sunscreen. Cancer teaches you how to find good in the murky mire of negative possibilities and to accept the small graces and minor mercies. There's a small, but very dedicated, group of you whose names come up on Facebook beside every "add a friend" suggestion I get. I hope you know who you are, and how much your five minutes a day is appreciated. When I began this, I was expecting to find the names of people I already knew each day, not people who were strangers prior to this endeavour. Honestly, I am somewhat troubled by this, but I don't dwell on it. There are people who have known me for years that posted one message, gave their five minutes, and let this pass from their minds. I could dwell on this, or come to the realization that it makes the work you guys do on my behalf that much more exceptional. Answering a call for help from a friend is expected, but answering one from a stranger is truly a Good Samaritan-type response. Your care and concern is commendable.

As far as the rest of the results go, here it is. The CAT scan I had on my birthday in May showed four brand new lumps in my right lung and four new ones in my liver. Additionally, the three active cancer areas in my bones all continued to grow. Only one of these lumps measured greater than 6 mm, but they all still concern me. I felt better knowing at least one lung was clear of cancer, because you truly only need one lung to survive. I felt better knowing that my liver was stable (in terms of the number of lumps) because a healthy, or at least functioning, liver is crucial for survival. From the first day I knew I had cancer, I said that if it wanted to take me, it would have to do it piece by stubborn piece. I haven't won every fight in this life, but even the ones I've lost haven't resulted in the winners coming back to gloat, because they already know how fierce the contest will be.

After three rounds of the new chemo regimen, I've been given another CAT scan. This scan showed that most of the new lumps in both my right lung and liver have been reduced in size, some to the point that they don't show up on CAT anymore. The cancer in and around my L3 vertebrae has been reduced in mass, and the accompanying pain has been reduced by radiation. I'm basically back to where I was two months ago. The chemo is having a positive effect, which hopefully will continue. Two months doesn't seem like much until it's a significant portion of your lifetime. Two months can be an eternity to someone in my position, and I am thankful for each day that can be given back to me. Plus, for a poker player, it's just nice to pull through on a one-in-five chance all-in bet. Turns out you can make money betting on this horse to pull through (for a while more at least).

I thank you each again for your help, your well-wishes and positive thoughts. I'll continue to look for new friends willing to pay ten bucks forward for good karma, and I'll chat with you guys tonight from Marsville. Have an awesome day.

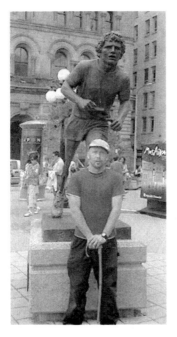

Two cancer warriors

WALL POST
SUNDAY, JULY 10, 2011 AT 7:08 PM

We just rolled into Ottawa. We're gonna find our campsite and settle in for the night. Tomorrow we go and egg Harper's house, visit the science museum, and then into Quebec. Have a good night guys, I won't have Wi-Fi after this, so I'll chat with you in the morning. And, hello to all our new friends. Take care.

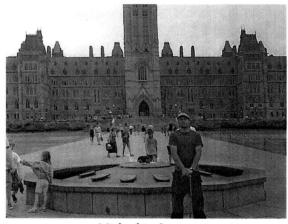

Michael in Ottawa

WALL POST
MONDAY, JULY 11, 2011 AT 10:54 AM

Gotta love Ottawa. My dad backed into a guy pulling out of the parking lot of McDonald's. The guy took one look at the damage and told us not to worry about it. His exact words were, "I'll buff it out." We dodged a bullet there. I'm off for a day of sightseeing. Take care guys. I'll send pics. Have a good one.

DAY 5 . . . WHERE'S THE F'ING OFF RAMP?

WEDNESDAY, JULY 13, 2011 AT 1:14 PM

Hello Facebook world. I'm currently travelling down Route 138 along the St. Lawrence, listening to the 500 Greatest Rock songs (according to Rolling Stone magazine). It's one of the most picturesque drives I've ever taken, filled with quaint little towns, big beautiful churches, and old stone cottages. There is truth to the rumour that churches, cheese shops, and gelato stands are in abundance in Quebec. Considering how often we've asked for directions, I've discovered there's no truth to the stereotype of Quebecers being unfriendly towards us Anglophones. Moreover, I've discovered that my attempts to converse in French have been met with smiles and amusement. We have discovered that it's still best to ask a male for directions, in any language. Sorry ladies, but we've travelled a few hundred kilometres in the wrong direction to validate this one.

Today was a much-needed break from the previous two days, which have been hard on my body and my father's mental health. Long stretches of being seated, without the ability to rest or nap to take the pressure off my back, is exhausting. I am, however, pleased that my father no longer owns firearms because he certainly would have let off a few rounds on any road larger than four lanes. Navigating through major cities really allows me to pause and question the way we choose to live (and I use the term *choose* loosely). It really got me thinking about the direction of human energy and ingenuity, especially with respect to how we live and travel, and the reasoning behind it.

Crossing from Laval into Montreal crystallized this question in my head. The sheer mass of people crammed into such a relatively small space really messed with my head. I am well aware that I'm mostly a country boy whose mind is dominated by small town ideals. As we crossed into Montreal, I wondered if anyone could find the key to open this sardine can. Then I realized that we've buried it under a billion tons of concrete and reinforced steel. We've devoted a lot of our physical and financial resources towards transporting ourselves from our homes in the suburbs to offices in the city. Our addiction to automobiles and over-consumption of fossil fuels couldn't be more apparent than on this section of the road trip. I marvel at the extreme engineering, manpower, specialized machinery, and dispensation of billions of dollars. We are almost always able to find an answer as to *how*. What eludes me is why we spend so little time answering *why*. Have we accomplished these things to make our lives more pleasant or meaningful, or have we done so just to facilitate the ease and expediency of industry? We travel for hours at breakneck speeds, racing between work and home. Observing a beautiful young East Indian woman blow by us at a buck-forty in a Kia, talking on her cell phone, with a *Baby on Board* sign in her back window made me pause for this consideration. Our priorities are definitely askew in the modern age. If our ancestors saw how we live and work, they wouldn't be amazed at the *how*, but I believe they would hold us to account for the *why*. Travelling through the outskirts of any large city, one notices the massive amount of track or row-housing complexes being built. The promise of a home (nearly, but not quite identical to the neighbour's) in the right neighbourhood is a lure for many, and an unavoidable necessity for most. Please don't take this the wrong way; we're hardly building slums here. We're building homes and condos of ever-increasing cost, despite ever-decreasing future value. And we're packing them in so close together that we'll never find the key to this sardine can. My good friend, Eddie, posted a news report on Facebook a while back, detailing the efforts of Japanese scientists trying to genetically engineer edible meat-like substances with what basically amounted to human waste matter. This is another example of *how*, without consideration about *why*, or at least *why not some other way*. It's honesty, not intelligence, that answers *why*. It is painfully obvious that we, as a species, would rather eat our own shit if it means we don't have to admit that there is a fundamentally better way to direct our path on this earth.

I have believed for years now that our emotional, social, and physical sense of well-being is tied very closely to our sense of identity and belonging. The further back you look into history, the clearer the lines of identity and belonging become. This also holds true for modern community sizes. The smaller the collection of people, the greater are the odds that each person will know and appreciate their place within it, and the greater the sense of overall belonging and purpose. When I'm travelling around in large metropolitan centres, I don't see this sense of place and purpose. I see professionals fully integrated into the rat race, others doing their best to not take part whatsoever, and an ocean of people lost in the middle. I believe that many of the physical, mental, and social problems we face today are inextricably tied to the way we live. Please don't misunderstand me; I still respect anyone who survives in such settings. I simply doubt one's ability to flourish as a member of a community that can't be fully identified. Whether it is environmental factors leading to physical illnesses or social factors contributing to mental illnesses, I don't see us living in a world that works well for people. I see us as another form of fuel to feed the machines, and there are a precious few that benefit from this sacrifice.

I realize I've gone off on a rant without any real direction here. Pardon the expression, but I'm just dying to get to the East Coast. I'm pretty sure I'll find a few people who are gonna happily owe me ten bucks. Take care of yourselves and each other, 'cause if you don't . . . very likely nobody else will.

WALL POST
FRIDAY, JULY 15, 2011 AT 8:54 AM

There is a town in New Brunswick called Beersville. This may require further investigation.

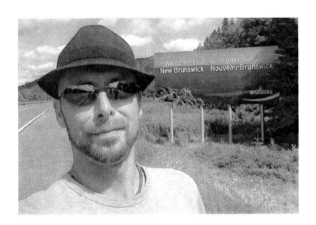

WALL POST
Friday, July 15, 2011 at 7:56 PM

We're in Shediac, New Brunswick for the night. We're going to Magnetic Hill, the petting zoo, and Hopewell tomorrow. Then we're off to the Confederation Bridge, which is the part of this trip my dad has been aching for. I'm off to check out the Irish Festival, and I may see Irishville tomorrow. Take care guys. I'll chat with you soon. I'm off to the festival.

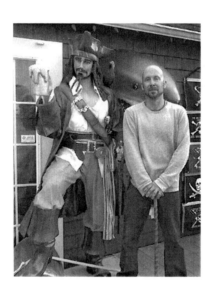

WALL POST
MONDAY, JULY 18, 2011 AT 7:08 AM

Good morning from beautiful PEI. We broke camp just before the downpour. It looks like it's going to rain all day, so we're going to watch the waves crash on the north shore, then head over to Summerside! Take care guys. Make the most of your day.

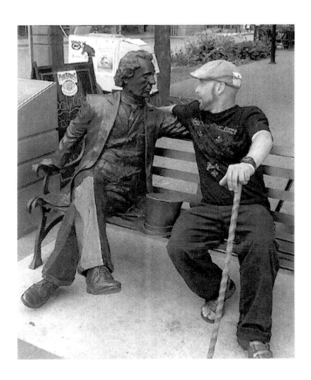

WALL POST
TUESDAY, JULY 19, 2011 AT 7:11 AM

Good morning from beautiful Halifax, Nova Scotia. I'm in the home of my old university friend, Shabazz Sallam. I'm going to go jump in the ocean at some point today and see Peggy's Cove. We'll figure out a way to continue on to Newfoundland afterwards without leaving ourselves stranded! The longer I'm on the East Coast, the less I think I would mind getting trapped here. Be in touch shortly.

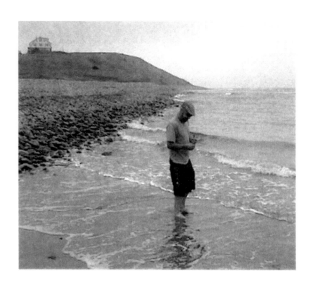

WALL POST
WEDNESDAY, JULY 20, 2011 AT 6:18 AM

Another good morning from Halifax, Nova Scotia. I get to go on a ferry ride today and I'm excited about it. I've never been on a boat where I couldn't see the shore. It's gonna be cool, and with all your guys' help it's gonna happen today. Thank you very much guys. I really couldn't have done it without you. I'll be on the road shortly, but I'll be checking in. Take care.

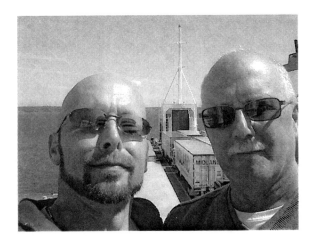

MORNING ON THE WAY BACK
THURSDAY, JULY 28, 2011 AT 11:23 AM

Good morning from Marsville. It's not much of a beach day, so I think we're gonna visit some mutual friends instead. It will be nice to rest up for a couple of days before returning to the grind of chemo. I have one more day of rest while my father visits his friends in Waterloo and Kingston. Thanks to everyone who's come along on this journey. It's been nice always having advice and info to work with. It feels exciting and sad at the same time to be on the home stretch. I'm already thinking of how to make the next big journey happen. Thanks again guys, have a good one.

ALMOST HOME
SUNDAY, JULY 31, 2011 AT 1:46 AM

We're just passing the Terry Fox Lookout, and then we'll be back in the Bay! Good night guys, it's been a blast!

MORNING . . .
WEDNESDAY, AUGUST 3, 2011 AT 8:06 AM

Good morning, folks. Apparently today is sunny (hopefully it will last a little beyond today). Lather up the little ones when you head outside and make sure you find something cool to do. I'm into day two of chemo. It gets easier from here on in. I decided yesterday to stick with it for the time being, in lieu of trying clinical trials out of town. I'll keep those options in my back pocket for now. I found out yesterday that Nurse Karen is leaving, but basically just moving down the hall, so I can still bug her when the mood arises. It's gonna be a beautiful day. Smile at strangers . . . it really messes with their heads!

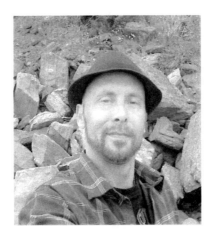

WHAT DOES IT ALL MEAN . . . ?
SUNDAY, AUGUST 14, 2011 AT 3:17 PM

Lately, I've been struggling to find my perspective on pretty much all aspects of life. This started during the road trip, shortly after the clutch fiasco, and has continued. Part of the problem is the way my mind is trained to work. I'm one of those (annoying) people who is constantly relating everyday, innocuous, little occurrences to the grand scheme of how the world now functions, or worse yet, how I believe it should be. Chalk it up to too many after school specials, but I'm always looking for the moment where everybody collectively nods their heads and goes, "Oh right, that's what we were supposed to learn here!" These moments are rare in real life, a fact I'm completely aware of, yet my brain continues to try to tie foreign concepts together, and place the entirety of existence in a concise, spiritually palatable, theoretical framework. Sometimes I annoy even myself, but most of the time when my brain does this, with varying degrees of success I find my perspective. I understand that often the end result is appreciated internally and is probably incomprehensible to most people around me.

I've been completely unable to take the first step in this process for the past month. The furthest my brain has managed to decipher its way through recent events in life is to identify what is screwing up my regular mental process. What I'm left with is a handful of things I understand with greater clarity and even more things with which I continue to struggle. I have always had difficulty in making my brain let certain things drop from active consideration into the background, clearing the flowchart in my head, so to speak. Anyway, here goes . . . What's screwing me up . . .

Where I'm at with cancer has skewed my thought processes in new ways. It wasn't until I received the test results, shortly before departing on the road trip, that I realized I needed to reconsider the direction and duration of my walk with cancer. Finding out that the current treatment regime is having an effect and slowing the sands of time wasn't news I was really prepared for. I don't expect to always have to endure the worst news, but I've learned that it's best to not be caught off-guard. It isn't exactly the first time I've received good news about my cancer. After the first two excisions were done, I carried the *I think we got it* good news for over a year. But we all know how that eventually turned out. Now, this little stalemate, my own personal détente with cancer, has given me pause for consideration. My brain doesn't know what to do with the time-outs between rounds. Since last July, cancer has felt more like a knife fight in the dark than any kind of comprehensible, remotely organized, process. I set my mind and spirit to stand against a process that I fully expected to increase in severity and complexity with a foreseeable end-result. I put my heart to rest with the reality of this, and prepared myself to lose everything. Now that the figurative phone call of temporary reprieve has come, I'm struggling to reorient myself to my new reality. Three months ago I thought I was the strongest I could possibly be and I was wrong. I'm stronger now, both in mind and body. My pain isn't on the same, constantly increasing path. My range of motion is returning. I can stay on my feet now for longer than I could before. I used to feel guilty on days when the pain didn't come, when it didn't make itself my alarm clock each morning. I couldn't process this guilt in any way that made sense, and now every day is like that. I'm not overcome with guilt, but the level of confusion is certainly challenging my mental coping skills. The closest analogy I've come up with is a falsely convicted death row inmate who receives a temporary stay of execution. Sure, it's a happy moment, but with certain, very tangible disclaimers that require consideration. More time can be a double-edged sword, especially when you think you've got it all figured out.

The road trip messed up my mental faculties more than I realized. Making the journey with my father was of equal importance to actually accomplishing it. You have to understand how my father tends to hold things inside, being strong for me and for his family, despite the fact that we worry about him not cracking up at least a little. Any tears my father has shed have been promptly put in their place by a stoic nature and adequate level of male pride. I wasn't much different for most of my life. It was the day we left behind the hurried madness of Montreal and began a very serene and peaceful drive along the banks of the St. Lawrence River that this mental haze really sunk in. For both my father and me, the trip felt like it really began at that moment. I needed him to see me at my best and worst. I needed him to gain his own perspective on this. We were both very comfortable with the scale and pace of life along the East Coast and appreciated the fact that some folks have really figured out how to live and interact with one another. By the time we exited the ferry in Newfoundland, the presence of a nearly untouched landscape had created more silent awe than conversation. There are many places we visited where we could have easily stopped and laid down roots. If someone offered me a crappy apartment on Water Street in St. John's, I would be writing to you from there tomorrow without hesitation. I got to see many people and places that I never would have without that trip. It forced me to reevaluate the way we (city-folk in general) live, because I saw so many people who have chosen to live in a decidedly different way. The general acknowledgement and care between people, strangers or otherwise, out East is remarkably different from what we were used to. I've never received so many greetings or head nods from strangers. I've never been called honey, sweetie or dear so often by women. I've never seen such hospitality or such authentic warmth in people as I did there. These amazing people made me consider whether I'm as much a product of my environment as they are of theirs. So much of how those people have chosen to settle the land and interact with one another made such great sense for people in general. This, in stark contrast to Montreal and Toronto, where every road is an artery feeding a city, filled bumper-to-bumper with trucks, whose contents are the life-blood of our modern lives of consumption, where far too many people, in far too small a space, are in far too big a rush to win a race that has no official finish line. I'll put it this way, on the East Coast, very few of the conversations we had began with someone tearing themselves away from a handheld device to grudgingly acknowledge the existence of an actual human being in front of them. It is truly a place where one's spirit can be restored and their faith in humanity rejuvenated, despite what the evening news would have us believe and fear.

I did say that I more clearly understood some things while still being very confused about others. I'm gonna get back to you with those in a bit: my head kinda hurts from too much abstract thinking!

I'm overjoyed to have made this journey and to have met all of the people that I did. There was a point where we almost had to cut it short. I am indebted to those of you who didn't let this happen. As much as my goal for all of this has been to raise money for people in need, I've chosen to do it by making people pay attention to what matters most. When purposeful and meaningful interaction with the people around you defines your life, it quickly becomes something that naturally happens. I am glad to have you guys paying attention to me and to one another, even those who are waiting to see how this turns out before parting with their ten bucks. I'll be back shortly to complete my incomplete thoughts.

PROUD TO BE A CANADIAN?
Friday, September 2, 2011 at 1:59 PM

It took four months for my disability claim to go through. During those four months, I exhausted all of my financial resources. I've been told I am not eligible for coverage for those months. If I wish to dispute this or the amount of my claim, my only recourse is a written letter to an office in Chatham, ON for reconsideration. There isn't even a way to speak with a person at that office. I was advised to apply to another program, Ontario Disability Support Program (ODSP), which also takes four months to be accepted. So what I learned today is that it doesn't help to have spent your life working hard and paying taxes, or how honest your claim is, and it sure as shit doesn't matter what your disability is. I've watched 20% of each cheque go to the government my whole working life. That same government is now prepared to give me $720.00 a month to live on until I die. I've been on disability for two months now and have been broke by the third day of every month after paying bills. At a point in my life where I should be eating healthier and have more incidental expenses than ever, I can't meet those needs. Something as simple as buying new glasses or paying for prescriptions can put me into debt. I've known people whose biggest problem in life is their fucking laziness, and I've watched them abuse our Welfare and Employment Insurance systems to receive greater assistance than I am getting. You can put the greatest people inside of a broken system and get no further ahead. I am truly ashamed of the system and the politicians who allowed it to deteriorate to this point — a point where it is better to be lazy and dishonest than it is to be dying and in need. Canada might still be a place where you can receive great care while sick, so long as you're prepared to die below the god-dammed poverty line when your time comes.

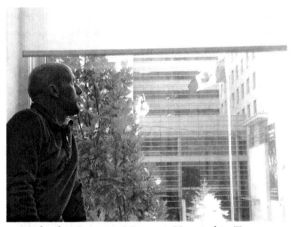

Michael at Princess Margaret Hospital in Toronto
Photo Courtesy of Hayley McLeod

THROW SOME DIRT ON IT . . .
TUESDAY, SEPTEMBER 6, 2011 AT 9:23 PM

It occurs to me that I've been a little short-sighted in my reaction to the CAT scan results. The last set of results was really positive and took me off guard, well . . . because I've never *had* any good test results up until that point. The results before that were horrible. But, objectively speaking, there are fewer nodules in my body than two CAT scans ago, and the cancer in my bones, specifically, hasn't advanced. The doctor actually said that there's been positive bone growth in my back. These are just the first results I've received while feeling better, instead of worse, each week. I did expect the test results to mirror what my body had been telling me. I think I just let one bad skirmish affect my view of the battle-at-large which, in many ways, I do feel like I'm winning. I've had lumps in my lungs and liver for over a year now, none of which have managed to take me out, and many of which have come and gone. As far as choosing the rest of the path from here . . . I haven't a clue yet. But I thank all of you for your advice, well-wishes and caring. It makes a tough guy a little misty-eyed to see the speed and strength of your feedback. I'm grateful for each and every one of you.

WALL POST

OK, just to clarify . . . I only have two pages on Facebook — my personal page and the *I Owe Michael Antcliffe ten bucks* one. The *Rest in Peace Michael Antcliffe* page, though well intentioned, is a little premature at best. I'm not sure who made it, but I posted a note to clear things up. I also found a relative of mine that I cannot remember ever seeing before. So that's kinda cool, but to clarify again, I just checked and I'm still alive.

GOOD NIGHT
THURSDAY, SEPTEMBER 8, 2011 AT 8:56 PM

It was a long-assed day and I spent too much time in the sun. I have an ODSP meeting tomorrow and all of the paperwork has been gathered. I ran into my old buddy Atilla. It was really good to see him. I'm gonna get his band to play at my fundraiser next month. I hope you guys had a good day. I plan to shower and make it maybe half an hour into a movie before I fall asleep. Take care guys.

Hey, there's a golf tournament in Pass Lake this Saturday to raise money for cancer and guess who got invited? I can't golf to save my life! I'm not sure if that's a double entendre, but it's funny on more than one level. 'Night guys.

WALL POST

My ODSP meeting couldn't have gone better. It reaffirms my belief that every process in life should begin with people meeting face-to-face and interacting meaningfully. It would have taken months of phone calls to accomplish what I accomplished today with a half an hour of face time. That's a load off my shoulders. That leads me to nap time. See you guys in a bit.

LEFT TURNS . . .
MONDAY, SEPTEMBER 12, 2011 AT 2:10 PM

The doctor's consult was a bit of a sudden left turn. As it happens, the current chemo meds are past their effectiveness. My options were not this limited yesterday. I need to spend some time educating myself about the available options, only one of which can be administered locally. I find myself somewhat stunned, because this is the best I've felt in months. I'm gonna turn my brain off with video games until I go to work at 4:00, then afterwards the Google classroom will be in session. I was prepared for this day; I just didn't think it would be today. I find myself missing those easy, seemingly inconsequential choices that make up everyday life. You know the ones that serve to frustrate and anger you from time to time? I miss those. At some point today (perhaps as late as tomorrow) I'm gonna have my moment. I've had it often and I imagine others have, too, but I like to think it's just mine. The tears will come and begin to flow quite freely. And when they are done, my jaw will clench and I'll swallow it down. My eyes will focus intensely as a wave of anger and indignation rises up inside of me. This will pass as quickly as it comes. And then there's the breath. It's like the one you take before you set yourself to a difficult task, a day of work, or a long journey. But it's the breath that brings relaxation, peace, and clarity. It's the breath you take just before you get on with it. I'll chat with you guys tonight. Take care.

FROM JANICE

I will start by saying that I read Michael's first note, *You'll Never Guess Who's Dying From Cancer*, back in April 2011 when it was re-posted by a friend. I was humbled, touched, and emotional when I finished. I quickly sent a friend request, as I knew in my heart that Michael was very special. I was instantly drawn to him. His eloquent words, and his ability to share his journey with cancer, provided a true epiphany for me.

I had the honour of meeting this brave, strong-willed, and determined young man at his first fundraiser at Galaxy Lanes, called The Bucket List Party, in May 2011. Michael's gentle way of making me feel welcome while facing cancer dead-on touched me deeply. I was awestruck just thinking about how much courage he had!

I shared Michael's story and his many other notes on my wall and am proud to say that many of my friends on Facebook joined in, helping to support his cause with eagerness. We continue to do so now, as we are all so very blessed to have Michael in our daily lives.

I follow Michael's posts daily, as he is always in my thoughts, and I love to read what he writes, describing his ups, downs, sadness, joy, and frankness with us all. He has made me cry, laugh, pray, and root for him in his battle against cancer. Being a very spiritual person, I believe that he will overcome this disease that plagues him.

The power of prayer, healing vibes, good karma, and strength-in-numbers from all of us combined, who have grown to love and respect him so much, leaves me to think that only goodness and healing will come for Michael.

The words *thank you* cannot cover the way Michael has opened our minds and hearts and made us look at life from a whole new perspective. The greatest gift he has given me is the phenomenal impact he has already made.

I am looking forward to being on his team, in June, for the Relay for Life. It is truly an honour to be sharing that experience with our team.

FUN DAY
Thursday, September 15, 2011 at 5:18 PM

I've been busy. It was a good day at work though. I earned myself a nap for sure. I have my next doctor's appointment on October 5th, so I have lots of time to do homework. Nothing is gonna happen until I speak with the melanoma specialist in Toronto. Regardless of what he says, I am heavily inclined to try whatever treatment is offered here, in lieu of travelling. I'll use the Northern Travel Grant if I must go elsewhere, but I'll avoid having to leave home if at all possible. Just like a kid, I'd forgotten how good it feels to have dirty work hands. Talk to you guys in a bit.

WALL POST

Morning Facebook world. I'm off for a few hours of light work, then homework, then something fun to do on a Friday that doesn't involve laundry. This evening's homework will be to educate myself all about Carboplatin/Paclitaxel immunotherapy treatment. Sounds interesting, eh? Not really: it sounds like science class all over again. I really have the urge to go see some live music this evening. Does anyone know of some good bands playing tonight? Talk to you guys later.

WALL POST
Sunday, October 2, 2011 at 9:53 AM

Good morning Facebook world. The original plan for the day was golf and dinner with the family. The new plan will be to head down to Emergency to get checked out. Over the past few days, the right side of my jaw has become tender to the touch and I've begun losing sensation in the surrounding area. It has hurt worse each morning of the last three days. I believe some x-rays may be in order. I'm gonna pick out a good book and head to the hospital. Talk to you guys later. Have a good one.

WALL POST
Sunday, October 2, 2011 at 1:26 PM

Well guys, no problems with the blood work, but the initial review of the X-rays shows something in the bone. We still need to see what the radiologist report says, but the doctor that talked to me had that *sorry to tell you this* look on his face. On the bright side, it turns out that I will make my tee time. I'll talk to you guys after many cold drinks and a few lost balls.

85

WALL POST

It was almost a complete waste of time at my doctor's appointment today. First, I found out that my body responds normally to basic neurological testing and my potassium levels are somehow high. There's been no word from the specialist in Toronto, and there are no plans to start any treatment without his consultation. Another set of blood tests and a CT scan of my head have been ordered. I'm sure the specialist will get to know my case by the first of next month because, if I don't have an appointment by then, he's first on my list of people to see when I get to Toronto. Balls, who wants to go have a few beers?

WALL POST
WEDNESDAY, OCTOBER 12, 2011 AT 8:38 PM

I barely managed to close my eyes, but I did get some rest. If I wake up tomorrow feeling like this, it's back to the hospital for me. I can't concentrate or function like this. Painkillers are only taking off the edge and dulling the sensation. The loss of feeling and the size of the lump on my jaw bone are both increasing. I can't feel my lower lip anymore. This can't continue indefinitely. I'll have to make some changes or do something.

WALL POST
TUESDAY, OCTOBER 18, 2011 AT 4:48 PM

Soooo, I have good news and not-so-good news. The radiation doc says that after a CT they can go ahead with radiation as early as next Wednesday. The bad news is that they need to do a cast mask of my face, so I'll have to lose the goatee one way or another. The tumour may have also caused a slight fracture in my jaw, which will require some type of minor surgery if it gets worse (see the original Steve Austin for details). And I also got my specialist appointment in Toronto for November 7th, so now I can familiarize myself with the Northern Travel Grant in all its glory. It will be months before my goatee grows back, which sucks because I'll wind up looking like some kind of cancer patient, lol. I've got a birthday party to attend this evening. I'm very much looking forward to watching a one-year-old face-plant into a birthday cake. See you guys later.

WALL POST

Good morning, Facebook world. I had an awesome sleep in my own bed last night. I had planned on accomplishing more today, but I'm off to a pretty slow start (just finished breakfast). It's time to start making some phone calls. And just as I say that, my doctor is calling me with test results. There are definitely cancerous abnormalities going on in the right mandible and the adjoining soft tissue. This isn't much of a surprise at this point, but it's good info to have before getting blasted with radiation. All of the funding for my appointment in Toronto is already arranged, thanks to ODSP and the supportive care department. Now I just need the dates for radiation. It would be a nice way to start this week. I'll let you guys know, but my plan is to be into full radiation treatment by the start of the month. I hope it all works out. See you guys in a bit.

WALL POST

MONDAY, OCTOBER 24, 2011 AT 4:05 PM

I missed the call from the radiation department. Man, it's really annoying being deaf in one ear. I can't imagine what people who are completely deaf go through each day. I'm really trying to get my next month planned out and I can't do it without knowing when radiation is. I'm gonna have to keep my phone on vibrate all day today and tomorrow.

WALL POST

TUESDAY, OCTOBER 25, 2011 AT 10:57 AM

My thanks go out to Lisa Laco, from CBC Radio, for coming to interview me and letting her listeners know about our efforts here. She's a very nice and sincere lady, especially considering how early she has to get up each day. She's going to air an edited version of my interview sometime in the next few days. She has also been kind enough to offer an mp3 of the whole interview, which I will find a way to post unedited on my page. Now I'm off to the pharmacy. I'll be back shortly.

90

WALL POST

I had such a good day today. I had a fun, fairly easy day of work. I also bought my plane ticket to Toronto. I will leave on the 29th (bloody early) and get back on the 13th. I'll have lots of time to visit with friends. Radiation will very likely begin on the 14th. I have live music to go see tomorrow, a shag at the Heritage Building the day after, and then I'm off. I'll have the laptop and phone with me, of course. I should find out how many people I can get out for a night on the town in Toronto.

WALL POST

Good morning Facebook world. I awoke today to a phone call from the doctor's office in Toronto, changing my appointment from the 7th to the 1st. Luckily for me, I planned to be there for two weeks, or I would be making a lot of rushed arrangements over the next two days. Doctors are just on a different page sometimes. I have a little bit of work to be done today, prepping and packing for my trip. There will be a bit of a rush over the next few days. Have a good one guys.

FIRST TRIP TO PRINCESS MARGARET
WEDNESDAY, NOVEMBER 2, 2011 AT 3:12 PM

I had the first of what will likely be many trips to Princess Margaret Hospital yesterday. For many reasons, I don't see how it could have gone much better. The hospital itself is impressive in its grandeur and modern appearance. Despite this, there are pieces inside that are both naturally artistic and spiritually soothing. It is very well-organized, both by its layout and the efficiency of the staff. I was trying my best to limit my expectations prior to my arrival, but I really feel no reason to do so now that I have been there. Everything I had been told about the service provided there has been proven true thus far. To start with, my only real expectation was to receive advice from a specialist as to the next logical step in my course of treatment. Beyond just receiving guidance, I was able to decide the next few steps in the treatment process. In addition, options that may have been on the table earlier have been removed or pushed much further down the list.

The doctor I met with was one of three that heads the clinical trial for Vemurafenib. Some people who have metastatic melanoma (cancer of the skin that has spread further into the body) have a specific genetic mutation called the BRAF V600E mutation. This mutation creates a protein that can increase the growth and spreading of cancer cells. The drug I will be taking prevents these BRAF proteins from working and thus prevents the growth of cancer cells. The clinical trials are already in their fourth stage. I had discussed this option with my oncologist in Thunder Bay and have already gone ahead and verified that my cancer contains this genetic mutation by having my excised tumour tested. The first step in the process was already completed prior to my arrival at the hospital. As with everything cancer-related (and most things in life), this option is a mixture of good and bad.

On the good side, and I really can't stress how good this is, the treatment is delivered in pill form. If you have ever received multiple I.V.s, walked around with a PICC line stuck in your arm for a week, or had to wrap your dominant arm in plastic wrap in order to shower, all in order to deliver medicine into your system, you can appreciate the value of just having to take pills. It's a huge bonus. Additionally, the effects of the medicine are felt by almost 80%–90% of people who receive it, and the effects can be felt within days of beginning the treatment. I will only be required to spend one day a month in Toronto and the treatment is provided free of charge, as it is a clinical trial.

On the negative side, this treatment requires constant testing and monitoring. One of the potential side effects is the development of non-cutaneous squamous cell carcinoma, the second most prevalent form of skin cancer. The fix for such side effects is surgical removal. Developing a less severe and curable form of skin cancer as a result of treatment may seem somewhat insane. But, with my level of advanced malignant melanoma, it's like telling a werewolf that they may develop rabies. All things measured in balance, it's a tolerable and acceptable risk. Also very important to remember is that monitoring skin conditions includes all areas of skin, inside and out. Women receive pelvic examinations in addition to the anal examinations that men receive. And I felt bad watching Molly get her temperature taken at the vet. It's gut-check time and definitely an occasion where it's prudent to leave all sense of pride and reservation at the door. Most importantly, the effects of the medicine have proven effective to an average of roughly six months. This may not seem like much, but I'm three-and-a-half years into a battle that statistics say I have a 10% chance of stretching to five years. If I fall within the 90% that don't make it five years, this medicine will have elongated my remaining time on this earth by 25%. That's a huge difference to someone in my position.

The medical team I met during my visit was exceptional to say the least. The doctor who examined me had an Australian accent and spoke with a confidence that bordered on cocky (anyone who knows me well understands why I appreciate this). He had a great sense of humour, and his effectively-used analogies emphasized his quiet humility. I was impressed that he took the time to evaluate and back up the interpretation of the histology of my original cancer excision and of the decisions my personal oncologist has made. What impressed me about the whole team of doctors was the amount of respect they paid to the lead nurse on the clinical trial, deferring to her skills and position as the *real* boss.

All things said and done, I was very relieved afterwards and have been impressed by the medical professionals involved in the clinical trials. I look forward to beginning the treatment within the next month and returning to Princess Margaret. It was one of those moments that one cannot help but be hopeful about. As with anything in life, time will tell, but I certainly feel like I have more time today than I believed I had the day before last.

WALL POST
Tuesday, November 15, 2011 at 6:21 PM

I just bumped into my neighbour, Archie, for the first time since I got back. When I asked him how things were, he responded, "All clear, it didn't come back." Archie's been all clear from cancer for about a decade now and, despite a recent scare, continues to be. I actually shed a few tears over the news (not in front of him, as men aren't down with that sissy crap). Last April, I would have smiled and nodded at the news simply because that's the on-cue, socially acceptable, autonomic type of behaviour that makes up half our lives. Last April, I hadn't even taken the time or effort to bother to learn his name. Today, I think I learned what it's like to be truly happy on someone else's behalf. It's a great feeling. I wish I'd figured it out earlier in life. Considering that both Archie and I have already cried in front of each other, something about this process, or perhaps all of you, is definitely turning me into a softie over here.

WALL POST
Thursday, November 24, 2011 at 12:00 PM

I just received a weird phone call from the head nurse from the Toronto clinical trial. She said that they sent my tumour to be analyzed for BRAF inhibitor mutation and it came back negative. That's weird because it has tested positive twice already. Even weirder, the nurse said it's possible for one tumour to test positive and another to test negative. The hospital has the original tumour from my back in addition to the one where cancer had metastasized into my lymph nodes. The nurse is going to make them do the test again, but the very outside possibility now exists that I may not qualify for this trial anymore. It's nothing to be too upset about, as I can still do another, but I kinda liked a lot of the aspects of this one. My fingers are crossed for a positive on the BRAF inhibitor genetic mutation (betcha that's the first time you heard someone say that).

LEVEL GROUND . . .
WEDNESDAY, NOVEMBER 30, 2011 AT 12:52 PM

It's been awhile since I wrote anything, aside from daily postings of this and that. I haven't felt like posting anything since my trip to Princess Margaret Hospital. It's been a few months since I felt like I walked on level ground, where I knew how much strength the next step would require based on how difficult the last one was. I was doing quite well with the last chemo treatment . . . well enough to be caught back up in the traps set by routine and necessity . . . well enough to go back to work for a few days and to enjoy my independence . . . well enough to become complacent and lose sight of the fact that this was, and still remains, a fight to the death. There aren't really any time-outs, just moments when that little place in the back of your mind convinces you that this isn't happening. My family and many friends also returned to the place where this wasn't a daily concern. We collectively slipped back into the routine of life without appreciating the fragile and temporary nature of it. We all began to do what I regretted most about my life before cancer, what I've been trying my utmost to demonstrate to others from my newly acquired perspective on life. We all went back to living day by day, without ensuring that we lived and spoke to one another like those days were our last.

Then cancer began to wake me every day with a little shot in the jaw that said, *Hey, remember me?* During my last visit to Toronto, my greatest concern and greatest source of pain was cancer moving into my jawbone and surrounding tissue. I had concerns about my slightly dysmorphic appearance and the fact that cancer was now within inches of my brain. I've since had radiation treatment on my jaw to decrease the pain and to bring the growth of the tumour under control. I've adjusted to not having feeling in part of my face. I've learned to stop biting the inside of my mouth into hamburger because I can't feel it. I've adjusted to a crooked smile and learned to check for drooling on the right side of my mouth while eating in public. I've accepted that cancer has half stolen the pleasure of a woman's kiss. When you step back and try to look at it objectively, it is utterly amazing what you learn to accept in the face of this disease. Realizations that at one point would have angered me to the point of violence get no more than a shrug of the shoulders now. To resign yourself to your fate is one thing. To resign yourself to the details of that fate is an entirely different thing. You don't get to be over and done with it. You need to check your gut each day. You need to ask yourself each day if the pain has become too much, if you can tolerate losing this ability or that bit of strength. Cancer doesn't just let you take the measure of your courage or endurance once; it comes back and asks you about it every single day. Through the pain, it demands that you answer.

I still carry hope and peace of mind that comes from having a plan of action. I'm still looking forward to the upcoming treatment decided at Princess Margaret. I do so because that was my last good day. The time before that, while I was still undergoing the last chemo treatment, I truly felt good. *Feeling good* is a relative term and the parameters by which it is defined change on a (near) daily basis. The time since then, waiting for the new treatment to begin, has been filled with a constant deterioration of my condition. The last time I was in Toronto, a lump began to form on my chest. I've already begun to feel the lumps in my lungs each time I cough, yawn deeply or even clear my throat. It's a pain that cuts through the painkillers and stops you in your tracks. It's a pain that sends your lungs, and entire body, into spasms if you can't control your breathing well enough. It's pain that puts a look on your face that will scare the living shit out of anyone watching it happen. But it was still pain I felt only if I coughed, or if I drew too deep a breath.

This lump forming on my sternum has taken the *if* out of the equation and now the pain simply *is*. It wakes me in the morning and tucks me in at night. It has taken most of my strength and mobility away. It keeps me in bed almost all day and makes rising from and returning to bed an effort in itself.

I've done more thinking about quality of life than quantity lately. I've gone back and taken the time to be angry, to feel cheated for all the years I will not have — something that I somehow considered myself above earlier. Despite the practice I've had, delivering bad news is something I really haven't gotten any better at. It occurs to me that I have more to lose now than I did when this whole process started. It occurs to me what an arrogant and hurtful thing it was to convince others to watch and to care. It occurs to me that I can always afford to smile and laugh at myself, because I certainly can't afford a moment of regret. We've arrived at the bumpy portion of this journey, I believe. I didn't put a lot of forethought into the consequences of asking you all along, but I'll thank you now for showing the heart to be here. I realize that it was foolish to expect level ground for any part of this journey, though it's exactly what many of you have provided. Two months ago, I couldn't have imagined how I would feel today. Today I can't imagine what I'll feel like in two months. But I *can* imagine how one should live in order to make the most of each moment, to live life with neither fear nor regret. Bear this in mind for those of you who are still asking your friends to come along. You may be asking more than you realize from them, as I have of you. Take care of yourselves and one another. This is gonna be one hell of a ride.

UMMM. ARE YOU SITTING DOWN RIGHT NOW . . .
SUNDAY, DECEMBER 11, 2011 AT 4:48 PM

I know, I know. Nothing good or happy starts with that line, but I'll make an effort. It's another beautiful day in Marsville; I had another great night's sleep and spent time in the best of company. I finished my fourth radiation session today. Upon my arrival in Toronto, I wasn't expecting any radiation at all. I was expecting to return home tomorrow. I was expecting that all questions about whether or not my cancer contained the necessary genetic mutation for me to partake in the clinical trial would be answered. I was expecting to be using the trial medicine and already be reaping its benefits. For these and many other reasons I've come across in the past few years, I'm pretty much done with expectations. Expectations, I've found, can be greatly built up and then dashed with a single dose of reality. Expectations can be basic falsehoods from their inceptions. Expectations can predict greatness and joy, and then disappear with the most minuscule amount of knowledge. Expectations, once they are laid bare in their essential nature, often amount to no more than smoke and mirrors. Hope, on the other hand, I have found to be far more durable and resilient. Hope is never false when had with good intentions. Hope flies in the face of reality and often in the face of objective truth. Hope can predict the return of greatness and joy long after they are gone. So from here on in . . . I'm with Hope, my de facto wingman. We showed up together and we're leaving together. Because once you manage to find it, once you learn how to appreciate it, and once you learn how to squirrel it away for when you need it you realize that's the kinda shit Hope does for you. That's good for me because, medically-speaking, nothing I've expected has come to pass.

I began my time in Toronto this time with CAT scans to my body and an MRI of my brain. This was followed by a consultation with one of the Princess Margaret doctors (a place that continues to earn every bit of its reputation). I greeted the doctor by asking if I had seen him on the *Cash Cab* commercial. He laughed and verified it was. I've only met the man one other time, but his eyes and every bit of his demeanor made me comment that this wasn't a good news type of affair. He told me it was complicated. We discussed my various pains and the still-mixed results of the genetic testing. The hospital has positive results and the lab used by the drug company has negative results. The hospital continues to advocate on my behalf, but as long as the drug company's lab says negative, it is highly unlikely that the drug will be made available to me. I'm generally the first one to jump on the *evil corporation* putting profit before people bandwagon. But in this case it would actually benefit the company to make the drug available to as many people as possible. The social scientist in me appreciates that giving me the drug is a pretty big slap in the face to scientific methodology and is such no way to develop a life-saving drug. Still no word on how this part of the story ends. The rest of our consultation made this portion of the consultation almost a moot point. The CAT scan revealed that the amount of cancerous (I'm sorry, *suspicious*) lumps in both my lungs have doubled and some have grown. The suspicious activity in my liver has also doubled. The lung-related news I could have almost guessed due to how I've been feeling. The activity in my liver continues to have no major effect on my daily life.

The MRI of my head revealed that cancer has found its way to my brain, in thirty different locations. Take a second, maybe re-read that last sentence. Christ, I had to get the doctor to repeat himself for more reasons than the charming Aussie accent. Cancer is now present in thirty different locations in my brain. Cancer is clearly not on a stealth mission, but is instead acting more like the Canadian storming of Juno beach. Establish the beach head, press inland and continue the full-on assault. From top to bottom, from left to right, cancer has established itself in every section of my brain. As is often the way with cancer, the news gets worse before it really has the chance to sink in. The two largest spots in my brain are located directly to the immediate left and right of my brainstem. Cancer has maneuvered itself into an advantageous position where it now possesses the ability, in part or in whole, to turn me off like a switch. Thus, the ten days of emergency full-brain radiation. The entirety of my motor skills and autonomic functions lay in a very precarious balance. As has been the case from the start of this battle, no amount of forethought or preparation can truly prepare you for the news. This isn't even the first time I've been told I'm dying — I've understood this for almost two full years. I've often equated my situation with that of a death row inmate (minus the obvious flaw that I've done nothing to deserve this). I'm in this situation for reasons beyond my control. My sentence was set the moment my cancer slipped beyond the first stage. My time frame was established when my condition became inoperable. But now, my friends, I sense the hangman testing his gallows. Hell, I can almost feel the frayed splinters from the coiled rope making up the noose as it is placed around my neck. Now I understand that it's a last meal and thirteen short steps before all of life's mysteries can be revealed. The doctor even told me that if I had driven to the appointment, that I certainly wasn't safe to drive home. He offered me his hand in comfort. He told me to gather my family around to let them know changes were coming. I asked how much he won on *Cash Cab* (over $800.00) and he told me his wife wouldn't let him double up.

This isn't the first time I've had to give family, friends, and loved ones such news. Rather than relive it through each retelling, I called my father and requested that he tell the family on my behalf. Telling my father was difficult beyond words. Listening to his

102

voice finally crack, gulping for the breath to speak, hurt more than words can describe. As a child, I vividly remember being outside cutting firewood with my dad. I remember the chainsaw kicking back a piece of wood and biting into his leg just above the knee. And I remember my father cursing, dressing the wound, lamenting the loss of a good pair of pants, and then ordering us back outside to resume cutting wood. A very memorable baseline was set for exactly how much bitching and whining was expected among the men of my family. Call it cruel, or macho, or whatever, I have carried the lesson with me since, and my strength has never failed me. I've always left the *feeling sorry for myself* shit for other people. Now my family, those who surround me, and all of you are up to speed. Now there's me and my wingman, Hope, wondering where we go from here.

Honestly, hope is going to be a challenge this go around. I'm still working on getting past some uncontrollable outbursts of crying. As usual though, I've taken a few days to acclimatize myself, to search out my little piece of level ground. I've found throughout this process that Hope and Mercy often walk hand in hand, never at exactly the same time, but never too far away from one another. The cancer I have can take you out by your blood, breath or brain. The liver can lose its ability to purify or fight off infection, becoming septic or turning on itself. The breath can simply become too hard to draw. The brain can slowly or quickly shut down. Is it better to burn out than to fade away? It's better to turn off than to slowly and painfully succumb to infection, or to not have the next breath. It's a harsh realization, but the odds that I pass on without having to gasp for my last breath have increased. There's some peace to be found in that. There is no help, however, with my other hope of continued walking. No different than the rest of us, I have a fate that will be met. I remain hopeful that my legs stay under me, that I will stand and walk to meet that fate. I still hope to be the first guy who tries out the new drug that breaks the back of this cancer. The humility I've learned allows me to hope that something about my case, my cancer, even the medical examination of my cadaver, leads someone to learn and accomplish great things in the field of cancer research. I hope that our efforts here result in a greater scope and accessibility of cancer care and diagnostic breakthroughs that give us information earlier to save lives.

I hope that my words and this page can become a place, a community if you will, where people can come and share, a place where people can both give and receive support from one another, a place where questions can be openly asked and answered. I hope that many of you can find strength and solace in this, as I have. I hope for a greater appreciation of family and friends, and all the truly important things in life we pay attention to after the bills are paid. And of course, I hope we can still find a bunch of people to owe me ten bucks. When you really get down to it . . . I hope. That's it, that's all I've got.

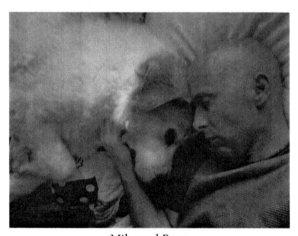

Mike and Roxy
Photo Courtesy of Hayley McLeod

FROM AMES
TUESDAY, DECEMBER 13, 2011 AT 10:02 PM.

All at once.
The world can overwhelm me
There's almost nothing that you could tell me
That could ease my mind
Which way will you run
When it's always all around you
And the feelin' lost and found you again
A feelin' that we have no control.

Today I woke my ass up at 6 AM and took a $16.00 bus ride from Montreal to Toronto to see my friend Michael Antcliffe (AKA Goater) . . . the poor kid has cancer. Yes I said it, he has cancer. As I write that, tears well up in my eyes, my belly cramps up and each breath is hard to take in. My friend is very sick and there is not a word, a thought, or anyone that is going to make that better. It's funny how angry I get at the people who say things like be strong, fight the fight blah blah blah . . . all of that bullshit. Clearly these people have his best interest at heart, but can you imagine how hard it is to be strong for all of these people when one is so tired. As I trotted down Dundas Street today to get to Michael, my teeth gritted, I was a little nervous. All I wanted to do was show up and just be there, not say anything, not even ask any questions. I just wanted him to know that someone who was strong was going to be strong for him today.

We shared nachos and cheese toast. The order went, "No black olives." The waiter graciously brought our food, covered in black olives, to the table. Goater sighed. He murmured. "I ordered no olives." I quickly grabbed the wicker basket with overcooked cheese and napkins baked into the plate and said, "This is not what we ordered." I was ready to beat the server. How dare he fuck up Michael's nachos! "Simmer down, Ames," I was told. I knew that it was OK and watched a disappointed kid pick off the black olives and leave them on the side of the plate. We chatted about the old *boogies* days. I tried to be two people, Ames and Pup (he couldn't be here). As far as I was concerned it was my way of bringing the two of them together.

Our nacho excursion proved to be exhausting so we went back up to the hotel and we lay on the bed (those of you who know me, know I have a boyfriend). Mike gave up trying to grab my boobs when I was 18 and I cut him off at the bar I worked at. I lay my hand on the tumour that has made a home over the midsection of his heart, the place that is most loving and giving about him. I realized that people who do not normally touch bodies can be scared of people who have cancer. The thought of breaking him crossed my mind, but then I remembered those big strong fists and the north end bar in Winnipeg, and realized I wouldn't hurt this guy. I lay my blankie across his chest, something else that rarely happens. It's my blankie and I do not share well.

He took shallow breaths, as though his nervous system was thanking me for holding him. The area heated up, we chatted and talked about I don't even remember what, but there was something magical around us. I held the back of his neck, cradled it like that of a small child. I tried to exude security, love, compassion, a few minutes of pain-free time. I wanted to take away all of his fear, just for a few minutes. I wanted to kick and scream, but the silence and stillness of both our bodies was just perfect. My hands were on his neck and his body was just lying there, getting some long overdue attention. Hope is not something I really believe in; I am a practising Buddhist and hope is something to strive for in the future. I believe it can sometimes take away from the moment. If we are always hoping for something, we often forget what we have right now. I placed my hands on my friend today, my friend that I love, my friend that I feel compassion for. I do not need to hope for anything because I know that in that two-hour period he felt something. We felt together — we felt relaxed. I love you brother.

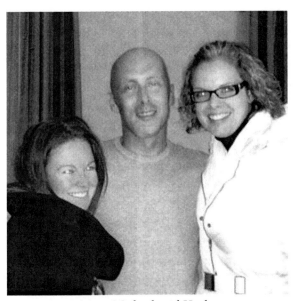

Ames, Michael, and Hayley
Photo Courtesy of Hayley McLeod

WALL POST

Good morning Facebook world. This is a morning that finds me more rested and in better control of my faculties than I have been for a couple of weeks. I'm going to spend a long day in the hospital with the hope that everyone gets back on the same page, medically speaking. The end result has been basically to give the doctors in Toronto some more time to advocate on my behalf regarding the clinical trial. They applied for an exemption to include me in the study, though the odds of it happening are quite small and another type of treatment, available locally, seems more likely. I have faith in the Princess Margaret team. The urgency and complete care approach they have taken over this last week was impressive. It turns out that the steroids I was taking also gave me a thrush infection, which antibiotics should deal with. I am due to return to Toronto to receive Gamma Knife radiation for a few of the tumours in my brain. I was lucky enough to squeeze myself in to receive radiation to my sternum lump, possibly before Christmas, but definitely before New Year's. My appointment is at 11 AM today. I kinda have that *just stepped off a roller coaster* feeling, and I plan to spend the remainder of the day finding my bearings. I still can't believe I'm going to see the Jets play in Winnipeg. The franchise left while I was living in Winnipeg and I was ecstatic to see that they were returning. Because of the level of fan support, and how quickly and completely the tickets sold out, I had resigned myself to the fact that I would never see them play again. I hope that karma revisits my friend, Mirco, tenfold and that the season's blessings truly come his way. I don't have the words to explain what his gift means to me. To everyone else, I thank you for the many shoulders that have helped me bear the burden of these past few weeks. My deepest appreciation and thanks to one and all.

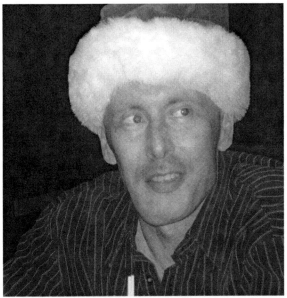

Michael enjoying Christmas with his family and friends
Photo Courtesy of Patti Stewart

MAMA TOLD ME THERE'D BE DAYS LIKE THIS, THERE'D BE DAYS LIKE THIS MY MAMA SAID . . .
THURSDAY, DECEMBER 22, 2011 AT 9:25 PM

I left the doctor's office the other day with a pretty distinct understanding of my situation and the required contemplations that needed to go along with it. I understood that the likelihood of my involvement in the clinical trial had deteriorated to almost zero. I understood that continued radiation treatment for the purpose of palliative care was still an option. I was also made to understand that the remaining chemotherapy option was moderate at best and carried with it the potential for hearing loss. I told the doctor that I wasn't willing to write off the clinical trial, as I believed that the team at Princess Margaret was advocating strongly on my behalf and it needed to be given more time. I began radiation to my chest with the hope of improving my upper body strength and mobility. I awoke last night with the ringing from my left ear having spread to my right for a full 30 seconds. I took a deep breath and snapped my fingers to assure myself that hearing in the right ear is still there. I really hope to have hearing in some form for the rest of my days, since I'm not nearly proactive enough to start learning sign language. Besides, if I lose hearing and manage to learn sign language, I don't know any deaf people to communicate with. It's another aspect or side effect that I need to seriously consider before starting the next round of chemotherapy. I'm two days into a three-day radiation cycle and I can already feel some improvement. This by itself doesn't put me much further ahead in the *where do we go from here* consideration.

110

I laid down to rest after radiation and was awoken by a phone call from a nurse at Princess Margaret. Not realizing until she dialed that I was rather far away, she explained in a somewhat surprised manner that one of the lead doctors on the clinical trial was requesting my presence at the clinic tomorrow. Somewhat surprised and confused, I asked for a call back from the doctor to confirm and went back to sleep. Awoken a few hours later by the doctor, continuing with the surprised and somewhat confused theme, he told me that the drug company had agreed to my involvement in the clinical trial after all. The team at Princess Margaret had applied for a waiver and advocated strongly enough on my behalf that the last available med-set of this stage had been set aside for me. Even as the words left his mouth, the doctor had a tone of disbelief in his voice. This medicine, which has an effect in 80%–90% of patient trials and lasts an average of five to six months, will be made available to me starting tomorrow. I'm on the first flight to Toronto (via Porter) tomorrow, returning the next morning. I had very little trouble arranging the flight schedule and the cost was the same as the previous airline I used, generally with two weeks' notice. So the reality of this day now is that the 'don't bet on it' clinical trial is happening and it starts tomorrow. Expectation, now set aside to make room for Hope, has won this day. A new chapter in this journey begins tomorrow. And, for once, I have news that I couldn't wait to share. Months of tears of sorrow will be replaced with tears of joy.

So when I speak of Hope, when I speak of actively looking for it, capturing it, cherishing it, and finally holding it close for when you need it, I'm speaking of days like this. I've had days where the sheer enormity of what someone in my position must be forced to contemplate has almost brought me to my knees. I've had days where I stare at myself in the mirror, am greeted with tear-stained eyes, and must remind myself through gritted teeth that cowardice does not run in my blood. I have had moments where, in the absence of any real thought or action, I simply break down, lamenting what is to come. I have had days that are filled with such exhaustion, such gravity of thought, and such pain that I would not wish them upon the worst of humanity. When I have days like this, I understand so much more clearly how it's possible to make it through all of those other days. It feels so good to give a bit of good news to the people you love. I have no problem hoping for days like this. I'm getting pretty good at it.

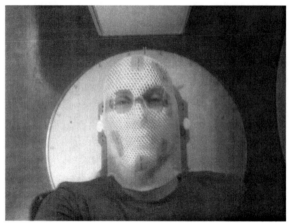
Michael undergoing radiation

WALL POST

I had a quick meeting with the doctor and he still seemed surprised that my name had come up. The pharmacist recognized the special order as soon as I put the prescription down and seemed quite excited, too. In 45 minutes I will have my drugs and will take my first dose this evening. This time yesterday the possibility of this trial was quickly fading. What a difference a single day can make.

WALL POST
FRIDAY, DECEMBER 23, 2011 AT 4:45 PM

I got my drugs; I got my drugs! On the paperwork under *How Does This Drug Work*, it states, "Vemurafenib harms cancer cells, causing their death." Sounds good to me! I'm off for a nap before dinner. Merry Christmas people. Have an awesome day.

WALL POST
SATURDAY, DECEMBER 24, 2011 AT 4:58 PM

Well, I'm awake after a nice nap. I awoke to our very own Lisa Laco dropping by with Christmas cheer. She brought gift certificates and the most perfect card I can imagine. The front is an over-the-shoulder view of a snowman looking into a stocking. "What's this? Two lumps of coal?" Inside is the front view of the snowman holding hands to his face stating, "I can see! I can see!" (lol). It's all a matter of perspective. Thank you very much, Lisa. I wish you and your family a great holiday. Mom has arrived and we're off to Galaxy Lanes. Merry Christmas Eve to everyone.

WALL POST

Happy Christmas Eve to everybody again. My family get-together was great. I've already fit in another nap and am waiting on the empty stomach time-limit for the new meds, so that I can begin stuffing my face with cookies (thanks Laurie). Santa can skip my place this year, because I've already received all that I could have asked for and more. My father and I will spend Christmas with family that we haven't seen during the holidays in years. I'll see my cousin Tommy for the first time in over a decade. Giving thanks and appreciating the true meaning of the season are things I can no longer just pay lip-service to, because now I clearly understand these things. This is my best Christmas ever, and I'm so very blessed and happy to share it with each and every one of you. So, hold each other tighter, let each embrace linger a little longer, and please don't forget the truly precious things in our lives. Memories don't come from under the Christmas tree. Neither do goodwill or peace on Earth. Merry Christmas everybody.

WALL POST
SATURDAY, DECEMBER 31, 2011 AT 2:50 PM

Morning Facebook world. Last night was the first ten-hour sleep that I've had in over a year. It couldn't have come at a better time! My mission for the day is to get some signs made up and go to the hockey game. My body feels like it wants to cooperate today. I hope the rest of you have had a great morning.

WALL POST
SATURDAY, DECEMBER 31, 2011 AT 5:04 PM

Well folks, I'm getting ready to clean myself up and prep for the game. I found someone with artistic ability to help with some signs. I also got an offer for reserved parking at the St. Regis, which is a huge help. I'm gonna get going early tonight, as I want to watch warm-ups and soak in the whole experience. With some collective good karma, the Jets should ring in the New Year with a win. Either way, I'm gonna have a blast. I'll be updating with pics from the game. Whatever everyone is up to tonight, please stay safe and look out for one another. There are too many other options out there for any drunk driving to be happening. Let's all have an awesome evening and make it safely and happily into the New Year. Go Jets, go!

116

WALL POST
Sunday, January 1, 2012 at 1:20 AM

Happy New Year Facebook world. I hope you are all safe and happily surrounded by friends and family. All other resolutions aside, this year resolve to be happy, to make a priority of family and friends, and to fear nothing in this world. Make 2012 the year you make your own happiness and question what you have taken for granted. I love you guys and thank you for the courage of walking this path with me. Peace!

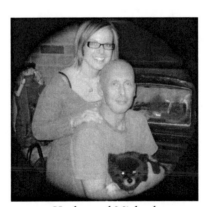

Hayley and Michael
Photo Courtesy of Hayley McLeod

WALL POST
THURSDAY, JANUARY 5, 2012 AT 2:40 PM

Let's hear it for sleeping in until a ridiculous time of the day. I woke up for an hour-and-a-half last night around 3 AM or so, and then slept until just after 1 PM this afternoon. Wow. I'm already running late for everything I had to do today, and I couldn't be happier about it. I should still try to get some of that crap done. I'm struggling between the choice of taking a shower and just heading back to bed. I'm kinda worried that I won't wake up 'til after supper if I do go back to bed. I had such a great sleep last night; I had forgotten what that felt like until this past week. Have a good one guys. I gotta get stuff done.

WALL POST
Thursday, January 5, 2012 at 6:02 PM

Despite a full night of sleep, my body is still telling me to take a nap, so I'm going to listen. Funnily, I've noticed the loss of 15 people off my Facebook friends list since New Year's. Guess I didn't make the cut as people narrowed down their friends list on Facebook. This does remind me that I still need to make efforts to reconnect with some of the original 134 I had before this all began. I'm not calling it a resolution, but I'll have to keep my eyes open for opportunities. The last New Year's resolution I made was to not make any more resolutions and it's been very successful thus far.

WALL POST

Ahhh, well it wasn't really a long day at all, but video games won over nap time, so I'm a little bushed. I'm visiting with my friend Nicole, taking my meds, and going to bed soon. My intention earlier today was to write a note to update you all and tell you about my trip. I have tomorrow off, however, so I'll have lots of time, and hopefully energy, to update you then. Here's the short version. It was a great visit. I stayed with a great family and met their family, too. The game was unbelievable. I found old friends, and the company couldn't have been better. Medically, things are not perfect, but this is the most *me* I've felt in over a year. I'm not a doctor or qualified to assess whether or not a drug is doing its job, but it's the only way to explain what's been happening to my body since December 23rd. So, tonight I'm fairly confident of my night's sleep. Sleep well guys.

MY HOLIDAYS AND LATEST TRIP TO THE PEG...
SUNDAY, JANUARY 8, 2012 AT 5:54 PM

In short, I had a great holiday season this year. I imagine that it was mostly due to the fact that I had a very clear head about what was important about the holiday season long before it began. I have always strived to avoid the consumerist pitfalls and materialistic desires of Christmas, and this year all I wanted to do was see as many and as much of my family members as possible. Being focused in such a way, I found it fairly easy to be successful. I managed to spend more real quality, face-to-face time with my family on both my parents' sides. Being able to see my cousin, Tommy, for the first time in over a decade was one of the best parts. Tommy is a highly trained member of our armed forces. In a time where the term *hero* is often misused or overused, I reserve using the term until speaking of people like him. When I speak of heroism, I speak of people who do more than act bravely in tough circumstances; to me, it's heroic to have *chosen* to be in those circumstances. The idea that someone chooses a life of duty, to have courage and camaraderie as their daily essentials, the idea that someone chooses to fight for their country and the rights of their countrymen, regardless of how tough that fight gets, is my definition of *heroic*. I could not be more proud that such heroism and courage runs in my bloodlines. I was so focused on spending time with family that I didn't think of much else. A side benefit to this focus was that any gifts I did receive, I valued that much more. A few surprise gifts and cards from friends online were very much the icing on the cake.

121

New Year's was unbelievable and memorable in more ways than one. The hockey game was more than I had expected or built it up to be in my mind (thanks again, Mirco). The seats directly behind the Jets' bench provided a view of the game that got me a step closer to being with the players on the other side of the glass. Hearing the coach encourage and critique his players, listening to the players talk and plan with one another, hearing the roar of the crowd or collective breaths of relief and anticipation provided some amazing perspectives of the hockey game. I loved how the Winnipeg fans sang our national anthem, but hollered at the top of their lungs when the words *true north* came up. I loved how Kessel and Phaneuf couldn't touch the puck without being booed. It was great to see fans chanting, "Leafs suck," but still socializing with the Leafs fans in a welcoming and friendly manner (I even saw a few Leafs/Jets couples wandering around). I was smiling from the moment I entered the arena until well after I left, making this an experience I won't forget. To all the Leafs fans out there, I'm completely aware that the Leafs won their next meeting. Stop calling, messaging, and texting to update me with such useful tidbits of information. I was a Jets fan the moment they returned and will continue to be 'til the day I die, at which point the Leafs will still not have won the Cup. Sorry, but these are harsh realities we all need to deal with.

Another thing that really made New Year's great was the people we stayed with. Brian and Cara are old friends of Hayley and new friends of mine. It was great to be in such a warm and caring household in a quiet town outside of the big city. While there, we visited with their parents. I found it refreshing that in today's very fragmented and distracted society that some families manage to remain so tightly-knit. To get two or three generations together at least once a week for a meal and a visit used to be something taken for granted, yet it was a hinge pin of tradition that most families adhered to. I consider my own family close, but the two halves of my family rarely intermingled. My immediate family can't seem to all get together once a month, never mind twice a week. It always seems that work obligations and schedules interfere. Without question, some traditions need to be strengthened and made a priority for families in general (mine in particular).

I said earlier that New Year's was memorable in more ways than one. Most of the other memorable moments came in the medical context. Firstly, my buddy Pete (who I lost at the airport), made it to Toronto, but checked himself into the hospital on the 28th. When cancer came back in his stomach, it cut off the blood flow to one of his legs and created a significant limp. Pete's the kind of guy I used to be and he tries to tough it out without telling people the kind of pain he's in. He lets things get pretty bad before he goes to the hospital and rarely calls people with updates. Both my father and I are worried that he's going to lose the leg and what his reaction to such an event might be. We're waiting for his call.

As far as I'm concerned, much transpired during the holidays. The radiation I received for my brain *sank in* so to speak and left some harsh tanning behind. The hair on my head has stopped growing and a fairly distinct line runs from the corners of my eyes to below my ear lobes and around the back of my head. My head and ears have fully peeled a few layers of skin and are just now starting to feel normal again (after many daily applications of coconut oil and cream). My eyebrows have been spared. For this I'm very thankful, because all of us know at least one friend who proves eyebrows can't simply be drawn on as a replacement or cover up. You either always look surprised, startled at nothing, or like some sinister evil genius plotting the world's downfall.

I've learned from cancer that one day cannot be judged accurately from the day previous, nor can it be used as a predictor of well-being for the days to come. I began taking the trial meds two days before Christmas. The side effects made themselves known quickly. Coughing, joint pain, and headaches dominated the next week, specifically in the mornings. Coughing felt like an ice pick to the chest because of the lumps in my lungs. Waking up to uncontrollable bouts of coughing was pretty hellish for about a week. The joint pain, which concentrated itself in my spine, was a harsh coupling to the cough. And the ensuing headache kind of blended the whole crappy experience together. I've been very careful not to assume the medicine is working or jumping the gun as far as predicting its effects. I was told that these meds are designed to kill off new cancer cells and provide some improvement of symptoms.

And then I awoke after noon on New Year's Day, fully-rested, with very little coughing or pain. The next day I awoke after 10 AM, feeling very much the same. Each day that followed seemed to involve some slight improvement over the day before. Still stuck in the cancer rut of not judging one day against the other, I remained skeptical and reserved any real judgment. But those types of mornings have continued, one day after the other, since New Year's. It no longer feels like an ice pick to the chest when I cough and the meds no longer make me cough uncontrollably each morning. The joint pain has gone away and the headaches are minimal at their worst. Then Hayley told me that the lump on my jaw was shrinking, which I didn't immediately believe (sorry baby) and now my jaw line has returned to almost normal. I had a lump underneath each armpit, one of which has disappeared almost entirely and the other is quickly following suit. The tumour on my sternum has decreased significantly in both size and sensitivity. A good portion of my strength, mobility, and endurance has returned. I didn't take any of my "take as needed" painkillers on New Year's Day and haven't had to use them since. My head may be a little toasty and overdone, but the rest of me is quickly starting to feel brand new. Even if these meds weren't killing cancer and prolonging my life, the quality of life it is providing makes the experience worth it. My appreciation towards the doctors who fought to get me into the trial has deepened greatly.

So, my holidays were crazy great, crazy enjoyable, crazy painful and ended with a crazy improvement in my quality of life and overall condition. For the first time in a long time, I'm optimistic about my next MRI results. I'm excited about participating in treatment. My brain is racing about the possibilities surrounding my next visit to Toronto, kinda like the way my heart races on about Marsville. I'll let you guys know how it goes (Toronto, not Marsville). I'm a gentleman.

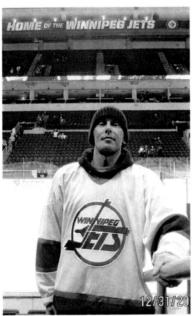

Michael at the Jets game
Photo Courtesy of Hayley McLeod

WALL POST
MONDAY, JANUARY 9, 2012 AT 8:40 PM

I had a nice supper and visit with mom. It's always nice when she comes over on the days when I'm most in need of direction and advice. I can't recall any major life occurrence or stress where I haven't gone to her first for consolation and advice on a course of action. I'm gonna try to stay awake until 10 PM. I really want to train my mind and body to sleep at the right times and get my schedule back on track as much as possible. I got all my medical paperwork done today but still have some things to figure out regarding the book and how best to make that happen. I think I may take a few of you fine folks up on your offers of expertise and organize a *meeting of the minds* in the not too distant future.

WALL POST

Well I got my MRI report back. It measured and identified 18 different lumps or nodules. My last scan showed 30, but I never did see the write-up on that one. I'll take it as a positive if 12 lumps have shrunken to the point where they can't be picked up by the scan. There's no way of really knowing this until the doctor examines the scans side-by-side. The Princess Margaret scans use a different viewer on the computer so it's difficult to compare. I really only have to wait two days to find out. I was hoping for something a little easier to draw conclusions from, but I'm relatively certain that things haven't gotten worse.

I got my new shirt and tie for a wedding I'm going to with Hayley, got my suit dropped off for dry cleaning, made an optometrist appointment for tomorrow morning, and got new sunglasses to replace the ones I left in the rental car. I found out that Dad waited too long to drop off his medical file and the nurse practitioner now has a full client-load. So, I'm off to the clinic tomorrow at noon to see a doctor with dad. He's resigned himself to the fact that I'm not letting up 'til he's taken care of it. I managed to get everything done that I had on my list today. I'm getting very anxious to get on a plane for Toronto. I'll have to nap on it for now.

WALL POST

I just saw a little girl with her family. Her shirt read, *Busy kicking cancer's butt again* with *again* in red and underlined. It's both sad and amazing how some are forced to develop such courage at such a tender age. Ha, she just walked by the other way. The back of the shirt reads, *Third time's the charm.* That's gotta be one hell of a tough little girl.

HUH, WHAT'S THAT, PARDON ME?
Thursday, January 26, 2012 at 2:24 PM

Normally when I sit to write a note it's because I have something definite to say, a somewhat formulated point to make, or simply need to do it as a form of release of built up thoughts. I think today definitely falls into the third category, so whatever you do, don't look for any semblance of continuity or a cohesive point here.

It never occurred to me that a return to normalcy and feeling like my original self would be such a difficult adjustment. I guess that adjusting to increasing levels of hardship and pain replaced what was once considered a normal life. The last chemotherapy I tried worked and did provide an improved quality of life. That still involved having an I.V. line in me once every three weeks and had a far greater influence in the form of side effects than this current drug has produced. I wasted that reprieve by attempting to return all of my life to how it was prior to cancer, not appreciating or willing to accept that the reprieve the medicine gave was temporary and not destined to last. This round of chemotherapy is no different in that regard. It is not capable of curing and its effects are finite in their duration. I am, however, determined to make my response to my body's positive reaction to this round of chemotherapy different. I am determined to make better use of this reprieve because I truthfully believe that I, as a person, have changed since the last reprieve and have grown just a little wiser.

I think the difference that has given me more clarity this time is my hearing or, more accurately, the impending lack thereof. You may recall that I lost the hearing in my left ear when cancer first returned as a lump in my left underarm. My hearing was replaced by tinnitus, or a high-pitched ringing sound. The whole process of losing the hearing in that ear took only three weeks. I vividly remember the emotions I experienced at the time, as they were inseparable from the larger picture of cancer returning. They can best be described as complete and absolute dread and fear of the unknown. I knew that if the lump in my underarm proved to be cancerous, that my formerly very favourable chances of survival had all of a sudden become a 10% chance of living just five years from the date of initial diagnosis. The necessary reorientation of the mind to adjust to this difference is immense to say the least. I remember checking my hearing on a daily basis and consciously keeping mental track of the volume and intensity of the high-pitched ringing. I clearly remember that day, sitting at my computer, when I was no longer able to hear the sound of my fingers snapping beside my ear. I vividly remember the feeling as the ringing took over, accompanied by an all-encompassing fear and dread of the unknown.

So, as it turned out, the lump was cancerous, my hearing on the left side was gone, and I was given no other choice than to confront the fear and the dread that were left. As we now know, the cancer has spread and, more recently, the ringing has also spread to my right ear. The ringing in the right has appeared sporadically over the last few years, or once every few months or so. In recent months I've heard it more frequently. Since the passing of New Year's, it has been a daily occurrence and, in the past week, it has increased to a point where it comes many times a day, lasting for over an hour at times. Now, when the ringing moves into the right ear, the range of my hearing greatly diminishes and the audible volume drops by at least 50%. I haven't a clue if the ringing will become constant, as it has in the left ear. I'm also clueless as to whether or not this will result in complete hearing loss, as it has in the left ear.

I'm once again staring down the double barrels of fear and dread with a background landscape of the unknown.

Only this time . . . I'm not afraid. This time there is no sense of dread. This time I am unconcerned about the worst of the unknown. This time I've simply put some thought into solutions and ways to get around the problem. I like to think that, back in university, I made my choices about what to believe and how to live my life. These choices have stuck with me since then and defined who I am and how I react to the world around me. Part of this belief system encompasses the necessity to live life backwards, to begin each day with acceptance of inevitability of my demise in order to truly behave fearlessly and honourably. Only in doing it that way can I try to behave selflessly and operate with an active social conscience. The transition from internally believing that you are fearless to truly understanding the depth to which such a belief can permeate every aspect of life was completed only after cancer, deafness, and other hardships presented themselves to me.

I cried when my neighbour Archie told me he had the all clear from cancer, and I realized that cancer had taught me to feel joy on behalf of others. I cheered when I learned that little Michael Michon and his family had finally made it to Universal Studios and I realized that cancer had taught me to celebrate the victories in other peoples' lives. I stood up straight and strong when my face and chest became infected and dysmorphic and I realized that cancer had taught me humility. I smiled from ear-to-ear when I saw that little girl wearing the *Kicking Cancer's Butt* t-shirt and I realized that cancer had taught me to recognize and appreciate strength in others. I began raising money and I realized that cancer had taught me the joy of giving without receiving in return.

Not so strangely, however, I feel the need to put true fearlessness at the top of the list of things that cancer and its accompanying hardships have taught me. I have completely loved only one other time in my life and that was quite a while back. I believe that it was fear that cost me that love and prevented me from appreciating its potential. Fear of making my heart available, fear of rejection, and fear of being exposed all robbed me of the full experience. This time around no such fear presented itself. This time around, the moment I heard those words, every wall and every defense mechanism that my fear had hidden behind instantly disappeared. This time it's the whole experience and it feels complete.

A man named Albert Camus said, "Don't wait for the last judgment, it happens every day." So from here on in I'm not going to frustrate myself answering every internal question. I'm not going to try and solve every moral mystery that presents itself. This time I'm not going to calculate or try to speculate how long the reprieve is going to last. And this time, I'll try not to wait until my mental faculties are bursting at the seams before I release my thoughts and share with all of you.

I'M WALKING TO CELEBRATE A REPRIEVE FROM THE WORST CANCER HAS SHOWN ME AND HUMBLY FOR ALL OTHERS WHO HAVE BEEN TOUCHED BY THIS SOON-TO-BE-DEFEATED DISEASE

TUESDAY, JANUARY 31, 2012 AT 2:07 PM

Last year I walked the Survivor's Lap at the Relay for Life, and it was my first introduction to the entire process. The event opened my eyes to the support, dedication, and involvement of some truly amazing people. The Relay is a real opportunity to immerse oneself in an experience that creates hope in the face of adversity. There, you will meet some amazing people and hear stories of courage, bravery, and survival. You will experience thousands of people coming together for the common cause of giving hope and support to those that need it most. Cancer can and will be beaten. It can happen in our lifetime, and it starts with people giving themselves to efforts such as this. I'm thankful for each and every day I have. I will be especially thankful when *this* day arrives and I am able to share it with my family, my friends, and my team. Agony of DeFeet for Cancer all the way.

WALL POST

Mom came over to visit today. She just came from having lunch with her sister and two friends they share from way back in the day. They were all getting together for the first time in years, having found one another after spotting each other on my Facebook page. I absolutely love hearing stories like that. It kinda tickles me.

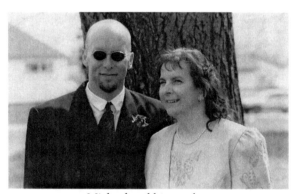

Michael and his mother

WALL POST
Monday, February 6, 2012 at 5:22 PM

I'm done with the hospital for the day. I got some good advice from a dietician for some tricks to try to gain some weight back. I arrived back home to find that things aren't complicated anymore, lol. Good stuff. The pain and symptom management doctor suggested that I try to lower the dosage of my painkillers gradually to see if my body still needs them. That was four days ago and I believe my body has given me the answer, so to hell with that idea for now. I need to change my diet a little, add in some foods that I've been neglecting, and get some type of exercise. That shouldn't be too tough. I also picked up the Pledge kit for the Relay for Life, which I will look through after my nap. See ya.

WALL POST
WEDNESDAY, FEBRUARY 15, 2012 AT 1:38 PM

Well, all is well on the medical front. My CTs on my abdomen, chest, and head/neck all show improvements. I'll still have to wait for the written report for specifics. I got my prescription for the next batch of meds. My doctor is already planning ahead for a time when this med is no longer effective. Things have gone as well as they could have.

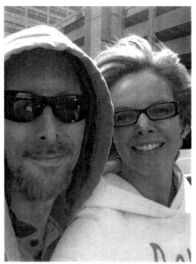

The face of good news

LIKE SANDS THROUGH THE HOURGLASS . . .
Friday, February 17, 2012 at 6:03 PM

I'm sure some of us remember the phrase, "Like sands through the hourglass, so are the days of our lives," from daytime TV. I'm assuming that soap operas aren't intentionally trying to be that deep and soul-searching, but I've thought a lot about time this past month. Not just time in the sense of dividing it into months, weeks, and days, but time in relation to all the other ways we measure it. It's difficult for someone like me, whose brain works in some very analytical ways, to deal with time in more abstract manners. It was attending Kazik "Bill" Pawlak's viewing that got my mind working on the problem. My first reaction upon walking in with my father was that we had somehow entered the wrong room. I took one look at Bill lying in that casket and every sense I had was trying to tell me it wasn't him. Clearly it was, but something inside me just didn't want to accept that. Immediately, my mind began to rationalize the feelings and gut-reaction I was having.

Bill was a vibrant person, very full of life. The energy he carried with him defied his age and, in a way, was captivating. I have memories of him and my father belonging to the same gun club and being hunting buddies. I remember sitting on his polar bear-skin rug and holding the custom-made gun he used to take it down. Apparently, Bill's memory of meeting me for the first time had me challenging him to pick out which one of us (my siblings and me) was adopted and which was actually born to my mother. Clearly I was young enough to be ignorant to the fact that he

137

already knew this information, but I'm sure he humoured me all the same. After many years of not seeing Bill, I only knew him through updates from my parents. Then one day, while I was doing a puzzle in the cancer clinic waiting room, out of the elevator stepped Bill. He took one look at my father sitting there and a look of authentic concern spread across his face. "Allan, what are *you* doing here?" He joked, "This is where people come to die." The look on his face changed to relief and then promptly back to concern as my father explained that we were there for me and not him. Bill began to question how I was and how my treatment was going, all the while ignoring or downplaying his own reasons for being there. We went to his home for a visit shortly thereafter. He was the same Bill I remembered from my childhood, with the same energy and quick wit, the same intelligence and strong opinions. Before we left, he insisted on giving us *a little something* for the gas fund for our upcoming road trip out East. Caring for those around him and generous to a fault, he was the same old Bill.

That's how he was the last time I saw him. Then we heard one day that he had gone into hospice care and saw his obituary in the paper the very next day; it all seemed like it happened so fast. It didn't make sense to measure the time in hours and minutes, mostly because there didn't seem to be enough of those. No matter how much you convince yourself that you've adjusted to the new understanding and reality that cancer presents, it somehow still sees fit to remind you that it's always present and waiting for you. Standing at the viewing, I couldn't recall the last time I had felt that mortal with so many details of my life, big and small, so very much in the hands of the gods. It reminded me of the first day I had to take my chemotherapy outside of the cancer unit. I showed up at the floor address on the appointment slip and found myself in the Inpatient Oncology department. Despite the fact that we're a bit of a rarity at my hospital, I found myself in the same room as another malignant melanoma patient. He was sleeping when one of his friends came into the room, looked at every person present and then asked me if I knew where his friend was. I was explaining that this was my first day there when my roommate woke up and greeted his friend. The fact that the friend didn't recognize him hit me pretty hard. It made me face the reality that this disease can change a person both on the inside and the outside, a reality later reinforced with radiation and the spread of my own cancer. I learned, in conversation with him, that he had the same cancer as I have and had been fighting it for almost two-and-a-half years. I learned that it had metastasized into his lungs and, most recently, his brain. My first thought was to ask why I was standing here, looking every bit myself, while he was lying there across from me, having become unrecognizable to his friends. It was a little over three years since my own diagnosis at the time. Looking back, it doesn't make sense to me to measure the difference between him and me in weeks and days either.

Shortly after cancer had moved into my bones, well over a year ago, I took a trip to Winnipeg. This time in my life was chaotic, and I found myself very much in panic mode. Learning that my cancer could no longer be successfully removed sent my mind spinning, and I felt as though things were on a short-lived downhill slide. I took the trip to go and say goodbye to friends that I felt I would never see again. Before I left I actually went through all of my personal possessions. I threw out useless things, returned items that I had borrowed, (cleaned the dirty magazines out of my closet) and took what I thought was the logical next step in preparing to meet my end. While in Winnipeg I sought out all of the people I felt like I needed to speak with one more time. I thought and behaved frantically, and it was very apparent to all those around me that I was afraid. That was almost a year ago, but it seems like yesterday.

While filling out the form for the Survivor Lap at the upcoming Relay for Life, I had to answer whether I had attended last year and how long I had been a survivor. Having been there last year as a survivor brought to the forefront of my mind that a big part of me had not planned on still being here this year. It became clear to me that, come Relay for Life time, I'll have survived this disease for over four years. It was simple math, but as I said, my appreciation of time is a little askew lately. It doesn't seem like four years. It seems like just yesterday and it has made me realize that I'd very consciously not planned ahead for anything because I had not expected to survive so long. I've certainly had no expectations in blocks of time as large as six months, let alone a year.

Without a doubt I feel as though I make better use of my time these days. I feel as though I pursue time with friends and meaningful endeavours more purposefully. I rarely do anything just to pass the time. However, I'm starting to realize that it's just as important to plan my life as though I do have the time; the same amount of time that anyone has to plan with and to enjoy. With that realization, it's easier to plan ahead to be part of a very successful team in the Relay for Life and to have a huge birthday bash, even though I didn't expect to still be here. I have time to meet some more people, time to contribute to a book and time to raise some more awareness and funds for others in my position. Most importantly, I have time to plan and have the same great people (and some new ones) in my life for a long time to come. I realize now that it takes toughness and endurance to survive, but it takes courage to plan ahead as though time were not my lifelong adversary. Easier said than done, but I'm getting better at it and all of you are certainly helping.

FROM HAYLEY

Cancer. It's one of the words that we all fear the most. It's a word that has affected us all in the most unforgivable way. We have somewhat acknowledged that there is no way around the possibility of you, or me, falling victim to malignant cells. We can all take preventative measures by living a healthy lifestyle and making choices that may, perhaps, decrease our chances of developing cancer. But the reality of it is that we are all prey hiding from the inevitable. When the predator attacks, we are in for the fight of our life. It is then that most of us realize how precious the life we have taken for granted is, and it is then that we embark on a new journey.

My world has changed since meeting Michael in May 2011. His heartfelt words of wisdom and veracity captured my heart so intensely that I had to see, for myself, who this man was. I spent a week in Thunder Bay, visiting childhood friends and getting to know Michael. There were many tears that fell over my face as he described to me the fight that he has endured. There was an abundance of laughter too, especially when we decided to go dive-hopping on a Monday night! This consisted of walking all around town, stopping at several bars (dives) having a few drinks, and moving on to the next. A couple of shots of Jack Daniels resulted in us becoming each other's leaning post by the end of the night. I awoke the next morning and ironically had the lyrics to "The Lazy Song" rehearsing in my brain.

Our friendship grew stronger on a daily basis. Michael quickly became a part of my family during his trip to the East Coast with his father, Al. They stayed at my home, and my parents joined in the company. It was awesome to see the connection and memories created in such a short period of time. Michael and I stayed in touch every day. It was as if I was right along with him on his travels. Let me tell you, absence truly does make the heart grow fonder.

Months passed. Feelings grew. Our desire to see each other became almost unbearable. We counted the number of sleeps until he arrived in Toronto (and still do) after each visit.

In December 2011, Michael arrived in Toronto for an opportunity to be approved for a clinical trial drug, Vemurafenib, which essentially harms cancer cells and causes their death. The doctor, a melanoma specialist at Princess Margaret Hospital, was very excited and reassuring that this drug would be an incredible benefit to Michael. It was amazing to see the relief and tears of elation on Michael's face. I was speechless. All I could do was hold Michael. We left the hospital hand in hand, with much hope and gratitude. It was comparable to Michael receiving a second chance.

Hope vanished soon after. Tests revealed the cancer had taken control of Michael's body. The number of tumours in his brain was beyond belief. I fell to my knees in shock. The clinical trial drug excludes those with brain cancer, and the doctor confirmed what we feared the most at that time — Michael no longer qualified for the drug that would give us more time together. Suddenly, the relentlessness of Michael's illness became apparent. The emptiness I encountered was more than I could bear. How could life be so cruel?

Ten days of emergency radiation began immediately. A couple of days in, Michael became more fatigued, and all I could do was hold him and comfort him. What more could I do? As he rested, I caressed his face and thought of each and every moment we spent together. I watched him sleep and imagined the cancer was just an ominous nightmare. I would lay with him, envelop myself in his arms and strive to be as close as possible.

On December 23, 2011, Michael called me in disbelief. The doctor requested his presence at Princess Margaret Hospital the next morning, Christmas Eve. God only knows how, but Michael was miraculously accepted to receive the trial drugs. I hung up the phone, cried, and jumped about like a little girl. Sleep was in short supply that night; excitement took over. Michael was flying into Toronto immediately and we were soon on our way to receive the most precious gift anyone could ever ask for at Christmas: time to love.

After only one week of the miracle medication, Michael discovered a new-found energy after a full night's sleep. This was incredible. We were visiting my best friends, Cara and Brian, in Winnipeg. We were gearing up for a hockey game that Michael never thought he would see: Toronto Maple Leafs vs. Winnipeg Jets. To top it off, a very generous friend had gifted Michael the best seats in the house, directly behind the Jets bench! Michael's reaction throughout the national anthem was a moment I will treasure forever. He was standing so proud, hand on heart, smiling from ear-to-ear, and his eyes were filled with tears of implausible elation.

Michael Antcliffe, you have conveyed a new significance to my life. I reminisce every moment you and I have shared thus far: our talks, cuddles, kisses, and heart-warming embraces. You offer the most eloquent embraces. I will, by no means, ever acquire a sufficient amount of them. You have helped me to understand the finer things in life and appreciate everything about the path I have chosen. You have given me strength to accept the things I cannot change and to change the things I cannot accept. You are my best friend, my confidant, and my love. Michael, you will always be in my heart. No one or nothing will ever change that. Same stars baby, for eternity.

I'll love you forever, I'll like you for always. Forever and ever, my baby you'll be.

~ **Robert Munsch**

WALL POST

Ihad mixed blessings waiting for me when I got home. The great part was my cool new toque. A huge thank you to Kathy, who arranged for me to get an awesome hand-knitted Winnipeg Jets toque from a soon-to-be Facebook friend, Stephanie. Stephanie has a page called Land of Yarnia (awesome name) that I hope you guys can all check out and like.

The crappy part was a letter from the government saying that my ODSP file was on hold and no further benefits would be paid while it was. Apparently, they needed to assess if I was still eligible and whether I was receiving the correct amount. I was instantly worried, scared, and unbelievably pissed-off. I finally managed to get my new worker on the phone, and she explained what had happened, including the fact that my file was fine, and not on hold. I went down to the office to hand in paperwork and to have my previous worker confirm what I had been told on the phone. So the crisis was averted, or at least taken care of before its effects were felt. But for a few hours there all sorts of scheming and plotting was running around in my head. Whew. Glad I took a breath and waited for all of the information to come in.

WALL POST
Monday, March 12, 2012 at 12:44 PM

It feels like it's going to be another day of sucking it up. My stomach is on the verge of nausea and I'm not quite sure what to do to lure it back into compliance. My head hurts and, worse, my jaw is starting to hurt, too. I never thought I would find myself hoping for a toothache. I'll have to see how the day goes.

WALL POST
TUESDAY, MARCH 13, 2012 AT 12:28 PM

I'm just getting ready to head into Toronto. This is the first time I've been on the laptop on in over a day. Thank you, guys, for all of the encouragement and well-wishes. It always feels good to have people in your corner. The side effects do come for extended stays sometimes, and it has been a pretty rough couple of days. I feel like I've gotten over the hump, so to speak, and feel much better today. The fact the sun is shining helps, but the fact I have to hide from it is a little paradoxical. I feel the need to win every day. I just need to remind myself to be humble and appreciate that just making it through, and drawing breath the next morning, is winning even if it doesn't feel like it in the traditional sense. Thanks a bunch for all you do. I'll check in with you later.

COMING FULL CIRCLE . . .
TUESDAY, MARCH 27, 2012 AT 3:10 PM

Lately, many things (foremost amongst them putting a book together) have led me to examine the recent past and hold it up to the present day's light. I put a dedication page in the book for my cousin and that led me to go back and look at his funeral page and all of the Facebook entries made after his passing. It occurred to me how present in my mind he was when I began this online fundraising effort, which will reach its one-year mark in less than a month. I've often tried to put myself in his place at various points along his walk, something I could not manage to do while we still walked this earth together. I find myself wondering what he knew, what truths he had arrived at in those days before he left us. I wonder if he had found his peace with this world, whether he left room for fear or regret in his final days or whether he had somehow negotiated an understanding of the process in its final all-encompassing nature. This type of thought leads my mind back around to the day I reached out to all of you and, in the midst of my frustration and angst, implored you to join me in walking this treacherous path. At that point I was visiting friends in Winnipeg and cancer had barely found its way into my bones. I was relatively new to the sensation of having my time on this earth drawn short, and I was in a complete panic and breakdown mode. I had spent nearly a full week with tears flowing and had begun to deliver good-byes to people I thought I would never see again. With the painkillers I was barely using at the time becoming ineffective, I spent a full day in hospital emergency being mistaken for a pill popper. The pain was so intense and constant that my breathing was affected and I began to feel weak and faint. I struggled to deal with sensations I had never felt before, very much believing that my choices had disappeared and were now broken down to *where* I would draw my last breath. At the time, I had room inside for very little, save anger and bewilderment. I survived with the help of a good doctor who took the time to listen and believe me. That night I began this fundraising effort. Since then, after sending out that first message for help, I have put myself on a path where rage and confusion no longer fit into the puzzle. Now, although the cancer has spread much further in my body, I have chosen to hold onto the peace and hope I've found along this path. In many ways I feel like I've somehow completed a circle without arriving back at my starting point.

I'm not sure the same holds true with other types of cancer, but with mine it has never felt like I got cancer just once. With the adaptability and mobility my cancer has shown, it feels like I've gotten it over and over again. I remember when I began to go deaf in one ear, feeling a lump grow in my armpit, and wondering what was happening to my body. I remember, after a peaceful day at work on a beautiful lakeside, dealing with the news that cancer had entered my lymph nodes; I learned that it had also aggressively entered my liver and lungs. I remember, after months of enduring ravaging immunotherapy, listening as the doctor described how it was very likely that cancer had progressed to my spine. I remember the look on another doctor's face as he searched for the correct words to explain that he would not operate on my spine because the procedure would not prolong my life. I remember offering up the clarification that the cancer had entered my bones elsewhere, allowing him to simply nod his head in agreement, both of us at that moment understanding the sentence that had just been laid down. I remember going to Toronto, so hopeful about participating in a clinical trial. I remember straining with every fibre of my being to hold myself together while the doctor described the formation of dozens of tumours in my brain, effectively eliminating me from said trial. Seared more deeply into my mind than any of these memories, I recall searching for ways to re-approach my family each time, responding to the hopeful look in their eyes with each new and harsh reality I faced. I remember the sensation of bringing such pain to the people I would have given *everything* to shelter them from.

Then I remember back to the very first time I was diagnosed with cancer, back in May of 2008, almost four years ago. Some part of me finds it beyond belief that I have walked this path for that long. It does remind me, however, that there is a story I once promised to tell you — the story of the first time I learned that I had cancer. The first step I took towards that revelation was to have a birthmark removed from between my shoulder blades. I did so upon the advice of a friend after some procrastinating and shuffling from doctor to specialist. However, after having the offending mole removed, I found myself at the mercy of a massive computer malfunction that affected the entire system of hospitals across the country. All test results were caught up in this massive information shut-down and people had to wait almost two months before the problem was solved. I, unfortunately, had my test results sent in right at the beginning of the mess and had to endure the full two-month wait. I was already back at work by the time my results became available. I had already spent a month calling an emergency toll-free number many times a day trying to get my answers, with no luck. Then, one day while doing renovations on the Dawson townhouses, the crew was having their morning break at the nearest Tim Hortons. I ended up getting a call from a nurse at the local hospital asking what date would be good to schedule a second excision. This was the first time I had heard about a second excision and I was more curious about the results of the first biopsy. The nurse on the phone, who was clearing a two-month backlog of results and appointments, clearly thought that I was already aware of my test results. When I expressed my confusion, she stuttered and replied, "Well, it's cancerous." Cue the Mike Tyson left hook to my midsection. I didn't make it three steps before I broke down, much to the confusion of the lady across the counter. I will never forget that the last thing I said before discovering I had cancer was, "large triple-triple." She probably won't either, lol.

I've always stopped short of thanking cancer for anything. However, the truth is that it has taught me many things. It has taught me both strength and humility that I haven't the words to properly quantify. It has taught me to celebrate the success and good fortune of others, regardless of my own situation. It has shown me the strength and courage in those I have chosen to surround myself with. It has enlightened me to the ceaseless giving nature of people toward strangers and rejuvenated my belief in the essential goodness of the human condition. It led me to experience love once more with the fearless innocence of youth. It reminded me that it is better to struggle and fight than to simply endure. Cancer showed me that hope can open doors, but it is faith that moves mountains. In my cousin's obituary, an often cited quote appears: "The man that refuses to stop fighting, even against all odds, could never be anything other than victorious." Well, I know my odds, and the only thing I know how to do now is fight. Only with this type of attitude do we have a chance defeating cancer in our lifetime. Success can be measured by nothing less.

WALL POST
Thursday, March 29, 2012 at 3:00 PM

I'm very excited to head to the border tomorrow. I can't wait to hold the first copy of my book. It'll be different when it changes from an abstract idea to something I'm actually holding in my hands. I'm hoping that everything in it is perfect, because this copy is going to my mom. Sleep well guys. Tomorrow holds great things (for all of us, some just need to look a little harder).

WALL POST

Book proof in hand and it looks awesome. So happy with it.

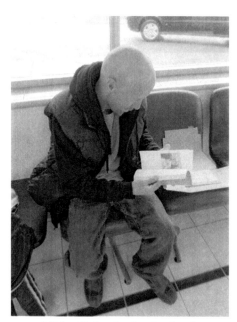

Michael's first look at his book
Photo Courtesy of Stacey Voss

WALL POST

Well, we had lots of waiting, with new and mixed results. It's kind of complicated, with not all things decided yet. Hayley and I are going out to eat and have a few drinks. The short story is that my meds have started to become ineffective. I have yet to write the longer story with the rest of my life. My treatment will change, but the journey will continue . . . as will I.

WALL POST
TUESDAY, APRIL 3, 2012 AT 10:42 PM

Well everybody, today was a tough one, no doubt about that. It was some tough news to get especially with someone you care so deeply about sitting at your side. But I've had worse news, and I've made it through tougher days. I'm still here. This isn't the first time a highly trained medical professional has suggested that I put my affairs in order. More accurately it's the third time, I believe. I'm still here. This is the fourth type of drug they've given me that worked for a while and then became ineffective. I'm still here. It is, however, the first time a doctor has come out to find me in the waiting room and stated, "Hey, I just Googled you. Good work!" Still here! Good night guys, sleep well. I plan to.

WALL POST

We picked up the first shipment of books and we're back in Canada! We were stopped, searched and questioned by the US border guards. The officer was rude and overbearing. He barked orders at me and was generally unpleasant. The Canadian side was the exact opposite. Either way, we got the books and they look great! I'm glad to be back on Canadian soil, too.

BOOK PRE-LAUNCH PARTY
Friday, April 13, 2012 at 10:32 PM

I had an amazing time at Naxos tonight. It was so great to share stories and hugs with so many people. It was an exhausting day, but it couldn't have had a better ending. Penny, thank you so much for hosting us. It was great to have so many friends and family around. Janice, your beautiful baby girl stole my heart away. I will keep her in my mind forever. This has been the longest of days, and I thank each and every one of you for your support. Because today's book sales exceeded our expectations, I'm hoping that people show up early at the book-signing tomorrow. I'm not sure we have enough copies left to last the whole day. We are, however, ordering more right away. Good night everyone, I'm wishing you all inner peace and good karma. See you tomorrow.

BOOK LAUNCH
SATURDAY, APRIL 14, 2012 AT 2:24 PM

Well, the rush is done and all of the books are gone. Today was a bit of an endurance race. Soooo happy to see so many faces, both new and old. Never underestimate how Thunder Bay comes out to support one of its own. I met great people today and made great connections. It's been a lovely whirlwind of a day. Thanks so much to all of you; my heart is humbled.

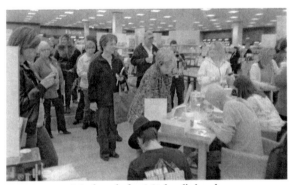

Mad rush for Michael's book

WALL POST

Tonight I'm signing off early. I missed my nap today and have lots to do before catching my flight tomorrow. It's been nice hearing from so many of you over the last few days. It's nice to hear the effect I've been able to have in getting people closer together. I wish you all a good night's sleep. My body is tired, my brain is still here, but my heart's already in Marsville. 'Til tomorrow . . .

WALL POST

Wow, obviously I need to pick it up with checking my page. There are lots of messages that will have to wait until tonight, as I'm still getting ready to head to Toronto. I hear it's a beautiful day there. Thanks for keeping tabs on me guys; it's nice to feel wanted. My flight is at 4:20, and I'm hoping to locate Pete within the next few days. I'm working on another book signing somewhere else in town and I'll let you guys know more as soon as it's set up. I'm also thinking ahead to a birthday bash next month; I could use some help with a location. I'm hoping to have bands, karaoke, and maybe a prize draw. Time to pack up the laptop. See you all from Toronto. Take care.

FROM KIM

Can you hear that? Please be quiet and wait for it . . . it's getting louder every day . . . come on, even the ringing in your ears can't stop this, Michael! APPLAUSE! Bravo, and take a bow my friend!

So, on the one month mark of my nephew Michael Michon's passing, I finished reading the book of my friend, who as we all know (or at least we should know . . . unless we are living under a ROCK) is dying from cancer. Yes, that's right, I said the word that no one ever seems to want to say! But it is real . . . just as real as every word of my friend who has shared his story with us all (strangers at first, but not anymore), his journey, his walk through the past few years of his life. Incidentally, I had no idea that this person, my friend, existed (other than by name only a short time ago) and last night I read the part in his book where he took the time to write about my nephew, Michael Michon. WOW! Words will never be enough to thank you for that.

Michael, it was amazing to meet you in person, to shake your hand, and to give you a hug, my friend!

For anyone who hasn't read Michael's book, you need to get a copy (profits from every book go to help people going through *their* cancer). If you really can't afford it I will lend you my copy, but not until after I've read it again!

WALL POST

Soooo, I got a little nervous when we were greeted by a neurosurgeon at today's appointment. The latest MRI shows a decrease in the size of all 30 or so brain tumours, including the three surrounding my brain stem. The only one that actually grew is located between the two halves of my brain. It grew from the size of one pea to two peas. As a whole, this is really the best news I could have received. It does the spirit good!

WALL POST

For those of you who might be interested, it was exactly one year ago today that this whole fundraising effort on Facebook began . . . with one simple message to a friend. Look at how far we've come now, and look how many friends we now number (eh, Nicole, did you know what you were getting into back then?). Love all you guys, old friends and new.

A NEW FORK IN THE ROAD
SUNDAY, APRIL 22, 2012 AT 4:05 PM

Well it may go without saying that the last month has been a bit of a whirlwind. With all that has gone on with the release of the book and the overwhelming response at the signings, I find my spirit very much rejuvenated. The next order of books should arrive any day, and I'm hoping to have another signing at Grinning Belly. I'm really looking forward to meeting more of my Facebook friends and supporters. It seems that the release of the book and accompanying news coverage has provided a wider audience and many new-found friends, which is always good news for the cause. The preparation for creating a non-profit is underway and the possibilities of that are both exciting and long lasting. I hope that we will create something that not only continues to support the local hospital, but also manages to fill in the blanks, so to speak, when other charities and organizations can't reach far enough. Many details have yet to be finalized, but it's uplifting to see the groundwork developing. Having the design for t-shirts done also brings a smile to my face. I'm happy to say that the planning for Bucket List Birthday Bash II is well underway for the latter half of May. The party will be held at Aden and will hopefully include bands and karaoke. This is particularly good news for me because, quite honestly, at last year's event I wasn't completely sure that I would still be around for another. I'm feeling much more confident about that now though. I'm also really excited that, in June, we will likely be holding the first annual Michael Antcliffe Laughs at Cancer comedy event at the Auditorium. I can't tell you much right now, except don't make plans for June 18th and be prepared to laugh your asses off at some great local and L.A. talent. Participating in the Relay for Life with a great team, which continues to grow, will be another highlight of the month for me. As busy as things have been, I don't expect them to slow down. I've really been working to get things organized before I begin this new round of treatment.

The results from the brain MRI the other day were very uplifting. I had no reason (nothing my body has told me, anyway) to expect much different from what I heard from the neurologist. The news was still happily received by both Hayley and me. In meetings with any doctor, with Hayley at my side, as she always is, I have the advantage of having been able to listen to my body and I usually have some general clue as to what the news will be ahead of time. Hayley, on the other hand, generally has to face the news somewhat blindly (an experience I usually try to either protect her from or prepare her for). The appointment last month with the new CAT scan results was one such meeting. I had a good idea that the medicine was failing, or at least that's what I thought my body was telling me. I did try to prepare her, but hearing the news from a doctor's perspective can still be overwhelming. What the doctor told us at the time was that the lumps located all over my body had, again, begun to increase in size without any real rhyme or reason to the pattern. My body had already informed me about this news. Although I still have an improved quality of life compared to the time before I started the medication, listening to my body had prepared me for what the doctor said.

Basically, over the last two months, I have felt old familiar aches and pains return to my body, along with a few new ones. Pain, or at least discomfort, is present in both of my shoulders all day. The rate at which my back becomes exhausted to the point of pain has sped up considerably. My mobility and my ability to lift or push things have decreased. The fatigue and tiredness that dictates my day's schedule has had its voice heard with much greater resolve. The lump in my right jaw has returned but has become two separate lumps — one on the outside and another larger one underneath. The outer lump has grown to the point where it seems to be loosening one of my teeth. The lump on the underside has gained a fair bit of mass and is only hidden by cutting my goatee straight across underneath it. A month ago I discovered a new lump just under the skin on my right shoulder. Last week I found another, again just under the skin, on the right side of my chest. Over the past two months, I have lost between 15 and 20 pounds of body weight. That's a concerning number for a guy who already started this battle very much on the light side. The last CAT revealed new lumps in one of my kidneys and in my neck. Perhaps subconsciously these past few months, I've resolved to work extra hard because I've realized that cancer is still working quite hard itself. In my eyes, a fight begins at the drawing of first-blood. I said to myself (and to anyone else who would listen) at the very start of this fight, just after the first excision, "If cancer wants to take me it will have to come for me piece by stubborn piece." To use old terms of battle, *no quarter given*, as I knew cancer didn't plan on giving me any. The plan remains the same, piece by piece. After doing some serious gut-checks in the last week, I find that my resolve has not lessened one bit. I still understand fully that only one of us gets to walk away at the end of this battle. I am more determined than ever that it will be me.

This brings us to the drug that I will start using tomorrow, Ipilimumab (Ipi). Most cancer drugs interfere with and try to stop tumour growth, often at the expense of healthy cells around the tumour. Researchers believe that some cancers escape detection by the immune system by shutting down antibodies (CTLA-4) before they progress. Ipi works by ensuring that this antibody is not shut down, allowing the immune system to remain more active and attack the cancerous cells. Ipi represents a unique approach to cancer treatment and isn't harmful to healthy cells. This is not to say that there are no side effects. There certainly are, and some can become very dangerous (even lethal) if they are not attended to in a timely fashion. Ipi requires some time before its effectiveness can be seen or measured. It only has an effect on roughly 50% of those who receive it (don't sweat it, that's better odds than I've had in many regards). The effects of this drug can last from a few months to over a year. I'm hoping to not only have the drug affect me, but also have the effects last some time. I've worked my way through all the most applicable drug treatments for someone in my position. After this I may have to get somewhat creative with my options. However, I'm not thinking after this right now. My mind is occupied with this current battle. The rest of the war will come in due time.

So there it is. The most complete update I'm able to give on all aspects of life, cancer, and how the two combine. I certainly don't mean to discourage anyone with this update. Life, with or without cancer, is a lot like hockey. It's great fun, moves pretty quickly at times, and it's always best to keep your head up, and your stick on the ice. Take care, friends.

FROM JASON
WEDNESDAY, APRIL 25, 2012 AT 10:00 PM

Hey Mike, I just got home from the Arctic last night at midnight. I was very happy to see the three books I ordered sitting on my table, just waiting to be read. Two of the books will be given away as presents. The first is going to a friend of mine who is a survivor and going through her second round right now. The second I want to donate to the Thunder Bay Public Library so that more people will be able to read and share your story.

Now back to the original message I've been trying to write to you since I first joined you on your journey. This is going back to our times at Churchill. It was in Sac's class and we were in the wrestling room doing some short bouts. I was, at that time, about the biggest guy in my class and not as fat as I am now. In you came . . . the little guy in the room . . . to show us some moves. I thought *I* was the tough guy in the class and here comes this scrawny little guy . . . and really, what's he going to teach me? Thirty seconds later I was on my ass, staring at the ceiling, with this scrawny guy on top of me. First: what a lesson in humility. Second: never underestimate the people around you.

When I was 21 years-old, I was diagnosed with ITP. That was the first time I had to be on meds and I discovered that trying to figure out my life was a test. I have been in remission for the past two years, after fighting with it a second time a few years ago. I may not be terminal like you, but when your body fights against you and leaves you laying there wondering if you're going to wake up in the morning . . . it makes you think.

Now back to that day in high school where you handed me my ass. It made me look at the world a little differently. So, while I know this message isn't really going anywhere, I had to say thank you for being you and tell you that really, you haven't changed much since that day you laid me out on my ass. It was just the first lesson you taught me. In the past year, you have taught me a few more. So, thank you.

FROM ROXANNE
MONDAY, APRIL 30, 2012 AT 2:53 AM

I've almost finished reading your book. It's been an emotional read and I've found myself sharing parts of it with my husband as he nods his head knowingly. Your chapter about your cousin and *my cancer* has hit home the most so far. When my brother-in-law was told there was nothing else the doctors could do for him, that his melanoma had progressed too far, I had the blinders on and got on with my life, waiting for the call that he was in the all-clear again. That call never came, but the call to let me know that he was gone did, and it hit me like a ton of bricks. I felt sick and ashamed that I didn't take the time to go see him. That will always be my regret. When I was diagnosed with *aggressive malignant melanoma* in 2009 (I say it that way because, honestly, those three words are the only ones I remember the doctor saying during that appointment) I still had my blinders on. So many people told me it wasn't *really* cancer. Even my oncologist downplayed it as something I should just forget about and get on with my life. That was nine biopsies ago, finding other precancerous lesions, so who knows how bad they would have gotten if I had listened to his advice.

That year, attending the Relay for Life, as I always did, they gave me a Survivors T-shirt instead of the usual participant's shirt and I felt ashamed to wear it because I only had melanoma and not "real cancer." I've learned a lot since those early days and wish I could do something to fight it besides earn the name Sunscreen Nazi from my friends. I've been blessed by friends who have gotten their

168

skin checked and a couple of them had issues caught very early. For that I'm thankful and will keep passing out information about melanoma. It *is* cancer and it *can* kill you. Thank you, Michael. Because of you, I know the names of most of my neighbours. We get together for BBQs, etc, and when my neighbour, Terri, was in a panic because her dog was sick and she was too new to the neighbourhood to know where a good vet was, she felt comfortable coming to me for help. I drove her and her dog, Kosmo, to my vet and he was well taken care of. Terri and I talk often now, as she is going through her own cancer treatments. In June, I will be hosting a street party/neighbour meet-and-greet where I will tell my neighbours about this wonderful man who taught me to reach out and connect with the people around me. And I will ask them to owe you ten bucks.

WALL POST

Morning Facebook world. I'm up even before the alarm today. I still find it exciting to go pick up books at the border, usually because it means we're out. I'm looking forward to the drive too. Have a good one guys.

WALL POST
FRIDAY, MAY 4, 2012 AT 12:05 PM

The books were picked up without any trouble. It seemed like a very busy day at the border. I'm dropping one book off for my Uncle Rick on the way back into town. I'm very glad that the next shipment is already ordered, because this one won't last very long. Thanks for all the support everybody. It does the spirit good.

WALL POST

Well, I've spent enough time waiting for my mouth to get worse. I awoke today with increased swelling. It's now difficult to swallow or to even speak. I'll take a quick shower, have breakfast, and then I'm off to emergency to get this dealt with. If my phone, which has been dying twice a day, holds out, I'll let you guys know how it goes. Otherwise I'll be in touch when I return. Have a good one everybody.

WALL POST
TUESDAY, MAY 8, 2012 AT 2:38 PM

Well, I've had pretty much every test they can think of done by now. I've been wheeled all over the hospital. The I.V. antibiotics seem to be helping (although that could also be the morphine). I get to see an oral surgeon eventually, I believe. I do feel better than when I first came here at least. Thanks for the well-wishes guys. I appreciate them.

WALL POST
Tuesday, May 8, 2012 at 7:52 PM

I need a damned credit card to get a TV — balls! Now my day has taken a turn for the worse. The doctor (surgeon) will be in tomorrow morning to see me. So now I'm allowed to eat, drink, and be merry. There has to be a lounge somewhere in this place. They've placed me in the inpatient oncology ward with my own kind, lol. Time for meds.

WALL POST
Tuesday, May 8, 2012 at 9:14 PM

Janice got me TV in my room. You are the greatest and I love you even more. It's been a trying day, and that makes it just a bit better. Big smiles!

WALL POST
TUESDAY, MAY 8, 2012 AT 10:12 PM

Being pissed off with cancer.

~ at Thunder Bay Regional Health Science Centre

WALL POST
WEDNESDAY, MAY 9, 2012 AT 7:25 PM

I just met with my oncologist, who was the only doctor left in this place I hadn't seen in the last two days. The plan now includes the removal of the offending teeth and *debriding* (removal of flesh) followed by some radiation. I will have to rush to Toronto for chemo and rush back for the 18th. It's gonna be kinda brutal, but there are no other options, really. Thank God hockey is on!

WALL POST
Friday, May 11, 2012 at 11:54 AM

It's official, I'm free. I have a few prescriptions to fill and some aftercare stuff to do and it's done. To everyone who sent balloons and such, your gifts were recycled to the kid's cancer ward, so feel twice as good! After a few errands I plan to have an evening of rest and visiting with family. Thanks for everything guys!

WALL POST

I was about to sit down and answer all my messages, then I turned on the laptop and saw how many there were . . . I'm gonna rest up a bit first. I'm feeling pretty good. It's nice to have a large bit of the necrotic-infected crap out of me. Thanks for all the well-wishes, balloons and messages of support, guys (not to mention all the visitors). It never feels like I'm in this alone anymore. Special thanks to Kim for carrying the book in her store. It's so great to have such support. Concerned about Stacey, and hoping her hospital stay is short and as painless as possible. Long story short, I'll still make it to Toronto on time for my treatment there. I'll just make it back on time for my birthday celebrations at Aden on May 18th. The theme is 80s and 90s Tight and Bright Night — hope to see many of you there. Come out and support more than one great cause. Thanks again everyone, I couldn't do these things without all of you. Peace!

WALL POST
SUNDAY, MAY 13, 2012 AT 7:49 AM

Another extremely painful morning brought to me by melanoma. Today it's mostly centred in my left shoulder, which is to undergo radiation shortly. On top of that, the clinical med's worst side effects have sunk in and now need to be dealt with. Don't get me wrong, I plan on having a great birthday. It's just that some days require so much more effort than others. Have a good one guys. If you didn't plan on a great day . . . tough!

WALL POST
TUESDAY, MAY 15, 2012 AT 8:17 AM

I'm up early again this morning with a little less pain than on previous days. I have to have an unfilled prescription sent down from Toronto and hope that it takes effect prior to my consult there. Otherwise, I may not be able to receive the clinical med. I'm not too worried, because the side effects have begun to retreat already. I also have to collect some paperwork from the hospital to bring with me for the doctors in Toronto. How difficult that will be, I have no idea. My stitches are beginning to dissolve and work their way out of my mouth. That's a little uncomfortable, but a good sign. It's not a horrible beginning to the day. We'll have to see where it goes from here. See you guys a little later.

WALL POST
FRIDAY, MAY 18, 2012 AT 10:32 PM

So it's 10:30 PM at my birthday celebration and I'm ready for bed. There was too much exhaustion and pain to overcome with today's rest. I'm gonna try to make it 'til 11:00, but I'll make no promises. Thanks to everybody who came out. Sleep tight to everybody else.

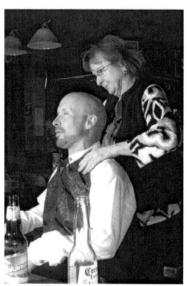

Michael and his mother at his birthday
Photo Courtesy of Teri Antcliffe

WALL POST
SATURDAY, MAY 19, 2012 AT 9:24 AM

Morning Facebook world. I had a good sleep last night. I only woke up once and didn't need to take painkillers to get back to sleep. I'm having a slow and painful morning today, though. The only thing I have to do besides rest is deliver five boxes of food to the Shelter House. Not a bad take for one night. Hope everyone had fun last night. I did until the tank ran dry. Have a good one guys.

WALL POST
SUNDAY, MAY 20, 2012 AT 5:46 AM

Little bit of trouble with this post, part spelling and part remembering. I managed to rest most of the day yesterday; I'm planning much the same today. Trying to stay relaxed in bed without expending any energy. Wish me luck. I'll still try to answer a few questions; you'll just have to give me some time. Thank you muchly. Take care and have safe days.

FROM SYLVIA
MONDAY, MAY 21, 2012 AT 5:10 PM

I was lying in bed last night and decided to pick up my copy of Michael's book, *You'll Never Guess Who's Dying From Cancer,* and let me tell you, I have a whole new respect for Michael and for life.

I figured I would lie down, read a few pages, and then drift off. It didn't work out that way. I ended up reading the entire book. And boy, was it an emotional read. From the first page to the very end, I experienced a roller coaster of emotions. It's like my entire cancer experience and all of the emotion, fear, denial, and anger came flooding back to my mind — all through the words of someone even more courageous than I thought I was.

I have been following Michael and his story for about a year now, based on a recommendation from a mutual friend. Jolene, I cannot thank you enough for introducing me to this gentleman. I read every note, status update and have tried to attend every event I could. I opened this book and the introductory chapter not only hit home, but also reminded me that I owed him ten bucks. Come to think of it, almost every chapter reminded me of that. Nicely done, Michael. I have decided that I will owe you ten bucks for every time you reminded me about it in your first book; let's see how much more you can get when you release the next one. Yes, that *is* a challenge.

I remember reading the note Michael posted about his trip to Toronto when he found out that his cancer had spread to his brain.

That day, I sat at my computer, crying for a man I did not know in person, but one I knew on a different level (if that makes any sense). As I read his book, I felt like I was going through every step of his journey with him. When reading the bad news, I felt it in my heart. The good news brought me joy. I laid there thinking, *wow, how come I never experienced any of this when they told me I had cancer?* I realized that during my own journey I was angry, downright pissed off, if you will. I thought, *how the hell does this happen?* I went to chemo and radiation, acting like it was just another doctor's appointment. I ignored the vomiting, ignored the pain, ignored the hair loss. I worked every day and pretended that there was nothing wrong. I did this not once, but three times. I never cried, but that was because I couldn't get past the denial stage. So here I lay, once again bawling for a man I do not really know, yet feeling closer to him every moment. I managed to get through the entire book, trying unsuccessfully to hold back the tears that continued to stream down my cheeks. At least that was the case until I got to the chapter entitled *From Hayley*. That is where I found myself bawling uncontrollably, not knowing why. Then I understood. The thing that I had needed the most when I was going through my own journey was support, but it was the one thing I was without, for the most part anyway. Not that I couldn't have had it, but I was so stubborn that I didn't want it and thought I didn't need it. Hayley spoke of *conveying a new significance to life* and those words touched me to my core. It was at that paragraph that I realized how much people take things like kisses, hugs, and even simple conversation for granted, and there are so many other things most people do not think twice about. Pleasures, like sitting in the same room with someone you care about and just smiling at one another or the innocent laughter you share between you when you realize how long you have been gazing at each other without so much as blinking. These pleasures are forgotten or ignored. I will be the first to admit that I take a lot for granted, even after experiencing cancer myself. After reading Michael's book, I vowed to change that. It certainly won't happen overnight, but I will do it in small steps so I do it right.

Hayley, thank you for your contribution to Michael's book. Thank you for the tears and for the realization that my life needed changing. Thanks for sharing your thoughts and feelings with the world. And finally, thank you for the love you shared with this incredible man. The world would be a much better place if it was filled with more people just like you. You speak so selflessly and it's beautiful beyond words.

Michael, you are one of the greatest men I have ever had the pleasure of knowing. Your outlook on life, the changes you have made, and the man you have become have made this world a better place. You may not realize it now, but you have changed a lot of lives and greatly impacted a lot of people. Not only has your book and your friendship made me a better person, but it has also made me realize that I need to make some changes in my own life as well. The things you are doing for the greater good are astounding and I hope the world recognizes your efforts. I pray every day that they find a cure for cancer and I pray every day for you. The young woman who lost her seven-year-old to cancer last year is a childhood friend of mine. I followed her story as well. I shared the suffering and the pain she felt. Too many people are being taken by a disease we have no control over; innocent children, men, women, and even animals are being taken by something that no one seems to be able to get a grasp on. I guess what I am trying to say is thank you. Thank you for changing my life and making me realize that I take too much for granted. Thank you for sharing your story and for touching people's lives. Thank you for standing up and fighting against this terrible disease. And finally, thank you for everything you are and everything you have become. I hope someday my heart and my mind are as great as yours.

To anyone reading this, take a moment to cherish the things surrounding you and the people in your life. You never know what may come of them, saying you're sorry now is a lot easier than trying to say sorry to someone who is no longer with us. Love the things you do and the people in your life more tomorrow than you do today and follow that pattern daily. When faced with adversity, it is better to be surrounded by love than alone with hate and anger.

Oh, and just as a reminder . . . you still owe Michael ten bucks.

WALL POST

That was pretty smooth as far as zappings go. I saw our comedy night ad in the paper, and I hear it makes it in a couple times a week. I cut it out all the same with a smile on my face. I also signed a few books for a radiation technician, which also made me smile. I managed to fill in a cancellation appointment with my oncologist at 10 AM tomorrow, which means I don't have to wait for the pain specialist. I never imagined that the hospital could be the best part of a day. I get slow cooked pork and potatoes for supper, so maybe I'm speaking too soon. See you guys in a bit.

WALL POST
Friday, May 25, 2012 at 2:57 PM

It's good to be back home. I'm glad to have seen my doctor, received new prescriptions, and gotten them filled. I even had enough energy to go visit mom at work, which I always love. I'm impressed that I was able to stay awake and get my ODSP travel paperwork done. It's been a pretty productive day and, needless to say, I'm in much less pain now. The full benefit will come tomorrow. Now, I rest on my laurels.

WALL POST
Sunday, May 27, 2012 at 8:29 PM

Well, I'm back from my Relay for Life team meeting a little early. That's the most organized meeting we've had thus far. Everyone should come check out our yard sale on June 2nd at the Young Drivers office on Waterloo Street. I have yet to figure out how to make Dragon Naturally Speaking capitalize and, honestly, I don't have the patience right now. I'm going to take my meds and try to get to bed as early as possible. The last thing I need is a replay of last night. I wish you all a good night's sleep. I'm hoping that we all wake up tomorrow feeling a little better.

WALL POST

I'm up early again, but not feeling as bad today, probably a result of all the sleep yesterday. I had a very surreal moment when I awoke to my whole family and a Purolator delivery arriving at the same time. Sleeping six hours in the middle of the day messes me up. It makes my internal clock think it's night or even the next day. So, I'm glad Stacey not only fixed Puff (my Dragon Naturally Speaking program, but I just call it Puff the Magic Dragon), but she also reminded me about the magic behind magnifying my screen. I don't know how this morning is going to turn out, but time will tell. Reading my book review did put me in a good place to just fall back asleep. Have a great day everyone.

WALL POST
WEDNESDAY, MAY 30, 2012 AT 8:01 AM

Wow, look at that! I'm up at a normal hour. I woke up for a short while last night due to the cold. Someone had propped open the outer door to our apartment building and it was freezing inside. I got back to bed and managed to sleep the rest of the night through. It was a better night's sleep than I've had in a while. I forget exactly what I had planned to do today, but I'm sure there's something I'm forgetting about. I checked my phone scheduler, but that was no help. So, you guys have a cool day. I'm going to try to remember what I was supposed to do. Take it easy.

WALL POST
Friday, June 1, 2012 at 7:16 AM

I woke up feeling fresh this morning. I got up four times last night but had solid sleep in between. I have no plans at all today unless I get surprised by someone. I went to Robin's for coffee today, like every other, but today I dropped my coffee on the way out the door. I only had time to cuss under my breath and throw out the old coffee before a fresh one was placed in my hand. That's why I love Robin's and Thunder Bay!

WALL POST
Friday, June 1, 2012 at 7:27 PM

Well, today's CT was as quick and painless as possible. I'm back at home with family and I feel much better. I can see an intensified look of concern on all their faces. They are becoming more vocal about their thoughts. That's good and somewhat overdue for some of them. Everyone needs to make their own peace with this.

WALL POST
Friday, June 1, 2012 at 10:07 PM

Wow, today was a long day. It was another one where I spent most of the day in bed because I felt the need. Dad's birthday was great. It was nice to see his brother, Ray, join us for a while and it's always nice to see Pete return to town. I managed to participate in the festivities for quite a while. My brother Chris is having a tough time dealing with my deteriorating condition. He was quite emotional behind those sunglasses. My family did well and Dad had a blast. It's nice to see three generations together laughing and socializing, and today will remain among the fondest of my memories. Sleep well everyone. Hold somebody close.

WALL POST
SATURDAY, JUNE 2, 2012 AT 12:06 PM

The yard sale is going better than we expected. It's really busy everywhere and everything is selling. Very cool. The music is great and we have two pros cooking on the BBQ and serving drinks. Thanks everyone!

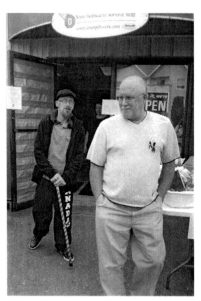

Mike and his dad at the BBQ
Photo Courtesy of Kimberlee Kirkup

FROM LAURIE
SUNDAY, JUNE 3, 2012 AT 11:13 AM

I remember seven-and-a-half years ago when we first met at the Brown Street Cafe. Your brother wanted to meet me but was too bashful (boyish-like actually), so he dragged you out so that he wasn't alone while he searched for me. If it wasn't for you, I probably wouldn't have given him a chance, thinking he was being a typical male in the bar. So, I want to thank you for being there and allowing me to know that he was just extremely shy. Then the holidays came and with that my best buddy at that time, Michelle Marie, came home. The four of us had such a blast that first Christmas and New Year's on Marks Street. I have so many pictures of us all during that time. Every time I look at them it warms my heart and puts a smile on my face. These are memories that will last forever with me. I am so grateful to have you in my life as my brother-in-law. Love you for always :) xoxo

WALL POST

Well, I got all my morning stuff done. I even got some grocery shopping done. I had to get my fresh fruit and Life cereal, of course. And I finally got around to answering my Facebook messages. It's good to hear from all of you and thank you for the well-wishes. I've been watching my Dragon closely and realized that he makes fewer mistakes now. I'm just warning you all, because every now and then he still says something totally ridiculous. It looks like it might take a little bit of patience on both our parts. I'm definitely going to sneak in that nap now. See you in a bit guys.

WALL POST
MONDAY, JUNE 4, 2012 AT 11:50 AM

Wow, I slept all the way through 'til 9 AM today. I was awake for a few hours last night, but the long slumber made up for it. It's time to shower up and pack my bag for my flight tomorrow morning. My brain is shooting off some mixed signals today. It's funny at some points, but outright weird and confusing at others. It's like I have no problem with walking, but suddenly I'll head off in a weird direction every now and then. Have a great day folks.

WALL POST
MONDAY, JUNE 4, 2012 AT 9:48 PM

Today was one of the weirdest days on the cancer trail so far. I had my ass totally kicked earlier by brain fog and confusion. I lay down to rest and slept nearly the entire day. I woke briefly to visit with mom when she came by around supper time, but slept the rest of the entire day away. I still feel like I can roll over and go right back to sleep. I should probably start packing the moment I wake up tomorrow. Good night guys, sleep well. See you tomorrow. Take nothing for granted 'til then.

WALL POST
Thursday, June 7, 2012 at 7:57 PM

I've had another long day at PMH and it began with me forgetting my pills at the Lodge. The hospital bailed me out, perhaps to make up for my chemo meds being created two hours late. It was a long treatment, but I was kept company by the whole McLeod clan. Afterwards, we had dinner at the Keg Mansion, which was great. Little Alyssa even interviewed me for her school report, which I'm sure will be very good. I had a really great day, and I hope the rest of you had one, too.

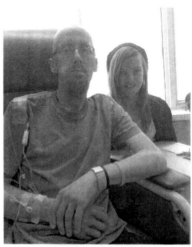

Michael and Alyssa
Photo Courtesy of Hayley McLeod

WALL POST

It's nice to get all of my messages returned. Puff the Magic Dragon is quite helpful, but I still think an eye doctor should be in my near future. There's only so much magnification one can use on Facebook. It's time to have the problem looked at. I wanted to thank you all for your words of encouragement. Words of kindness and praise are always appreciated, but I do need to be reminded not to try to fight this battle all alone. I need to be told when to reach out for strength and support, and there's a few of you who have no trouble reminding me. For that I am grateful and in your debt. I think it's time to lie down and see where my body takes me. Thanks for everything guys, I mean it. I wouldn't still be here without you.

WALL POST

It's time to test my eyesight and answer my messages. My decreasing vision is making this increasingly more challenging. Things have otherwise been fairly pleasant most of the day (I've done nothing but rest). We have a family dinner tonight that I need to rest up for. It's nice to see new pics up on Facebook, which is the only thing I can look at without magnification. See you guys a little later!

WALL POST
MONDAY, JUNE 11, 2012 AT 4:57 PM

All right. Everyone at once now — I fell in the living room around 5 AM and broke my right arm. I broke it right in between two cancerous modules, so I may lose a couple of inches off the arm. I appreciate all the calls. No need to worry; I'll be all right.

CANDICE POSTED TO MICHAEL ANTCLIFFE
TUESDAY, JUNE 12, 2012 AT 9:58 PM

It is with a great privilege, and at Michael's request, that I update all 4,644 of you by giving you a sigh of relief. I visited with Michael shortly after his arrival back in his room from the recovery area. His surgery was three-and-a-half hours long, and apparently everything went well. Unfortunately, he broke his arm right in between two tumours. The plan was to take the tumours out and connect the bone back together, either with graphing or metal rods and screws, but the doctors weren't really sure until they got in there.

He is doing well and was quite comfortable, generally speaking. His demeanor was typical Mike and he was even grinning ear-to-ear when I gave him a kiss on the cheek courtesy of "someone really special." ;) I held his hand and told him that we were all thinking of him and to not worry about a single thing. He did mention the Relay this Friday and I told him we are getting him there, no matter what it takes. He kind of winked at that. :) I didn't really get too much information about how long he is going to be stuck in the hospital.

I did find out that he tripped in the living room (possibly the foot of the couch) as he was heading outside. His father brought him to the ER right away.

Aside from looking like a typical surgical patient (somewhat stoned), his colour was nice and his movements were understandably slow.

His mom, dad, Auntie Teri, and I only stayed for 15 minutes and then we all left so he could get some rest. He asked me to update all of you and to thank you for all of your well-wishes and prayers. I'll ask you to keep 'em coming!

I hope you all can sleep a little better tonight . . . I know I sure had a helluva time last night, and he was on my mind alllllllllll day, as I'm sure he was on all of yours. I *had* to see him for my own peace of mind and to hold his hand and let him know that he wasn't alone. If I hear of any other new news or information I will keep you all posted as best I can (and of course at the kid's request). On behalf of Michael Antcliffe, I wish you all a good night. Sleep well . . . and don't forget to hug someone you love tonight and tell them that you love them, too! xoxoxoxoxo

CHRISTINE POSTED TO MICHAEL ANTCLIFFE
WEDNESDAY, JUNE 13, 2012 AT 8:24 PM

OK gang, I went to visit Michael this afternoon and he is doing well! In my opinion, he is doing exceptionally well, all things considered. He definitely still has his sense of humour. I say that because he asked me if I had time to help him get a bowl of cereal, so I asked him if he's had breakfast, and he said he wasn't supposed to, but he had some cereal (as he brought his own box of Life cereal with him to Emergency). I then told him that what they don't know won't hurt them and he agreed. He's hoping to get out of the hospital to be able to attend the Relay on Friday and the comedy night on Monday. What a guy! We're all worrying about him and he's busy worrying about everything else. How typical of him, though! Overall, he's in a really good mood and looks great, so I thought I'd pass that information on to you guys!

WALL POST
THURSDAY, JUNE 14, 2012 AT 12:39 PM

Just a quick message for you guys. I just got home from the hospital. It turns out the piece of steel in my arm is a little bigger than I thought. It took 38 staples to close the wound. I appreciate all of the well-wishes on Facebook. You guys are an unbelievable source of support. I appreciate each and every one of you — old and new.

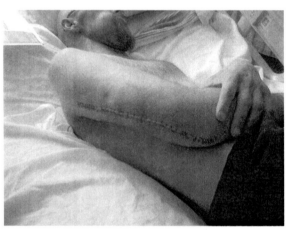

Michael's arm after surgery

WALL POST
Saturday, June 16, 2012 at 8:07 PM

Good morning Facebook world. Congratulations to my Agony of DeFeet team. Sorry I couldn't stay. I had a great sleep, though. Relay for Life was amazing. You were amazing.

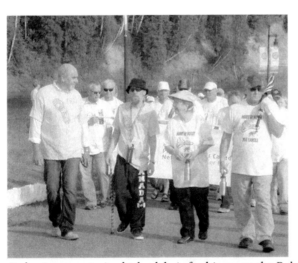

Despite having a motorized wheelchair for his use at the Relay, Michael insisted that he walk the Survivor's Lap. Seen in front: Thunder Bay Mayor, Keith Hobbs, Michael, and his mom and dad
Photo Courtesy of Candice Syrek

WALL POST

Good morning. I got most of my running around done and was called in to do some radiation I wasn't expecting. I hope it doesn't zap me too much for tonight's show.

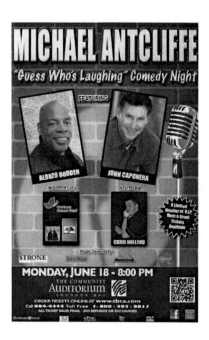

WALL POST

TUESDAY, JUNE 19, 2012 AT 12:05 AM

I've had another great night, great comics, great family — and world class friends! Good night guys!

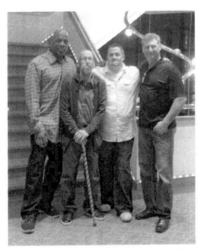

Alonzo Bodden, Michael Antcliffe, Chris Holland and John Caponera at the "Guess Who's Laughing" comedy night
Photo Courtesy of Jeannie Rempel

WALL POST
Tuesday, June 19, 2012 at 7:17 PM

I've awoken from a nice nap, but it feels like I've really only had half a nap. But, although it was a lazy day, I got quite a bit done. Not often do I have the chance to realize how little is actually on TV. It's a weird feeling, being able to exercise my right to choose something after feeling like so much of my time and choices have been decided by cancer. Something as simple as changing the channel can show me how much power I actually have. I should spend a little more time channel surfing without caring where I wind up.

WALL POST
Wednesday, June 20, 2012 at 9:16 PM

Good night Facebook world. I had a pretty good day. I'm going to see if I can stay awake for a bit of an evening (hopefully involving ice cream) with Michelle. It's probably wrong of me to have you all wish me luck. Sleep well guys!

WALL POST
Friday, June 22, 2012 at 3:00 PM

I've tried again and again. I cannot return my messages. I just can't read them well enough. If I couldn't type, I couldn't communicate at all. My body hates it when I sit in my chair to type. I cannot focus enough to capture the words. If it were not for the red underlining, this would be full of mistakes. I'll find something, get help, or whatever. Talk to you guys when I can. I see a little better when I'm rested. I will try that first.

WALL POST
Friday, June 22, 2012 at 8:43 PM

Well I've had a five-hour long nap. I was hoping my focus would improve, but apparently it didn't want to. Looks like I'll have to figure something out. I'm heading back to bed, likely for the night. I will be welcoming any suggestions (within my spending range) that don't involve animal sacrifice (large animals anyway). Talk to you guys tomorrow, hopefully.

WALL POST

It's getting 'round bedtime. Glad that hot and humid weather left before I went to bed. Except for packing, tomorrow is a rest-day too. I guess every day is, maybe from here on in. Stacey brought me a program that reads the text on the screen, so we'll see if my communication skills improve. Good night.

WALL POST

I'm finally off for a nap. The team at the hospital gave the OK for me to receive chemo tomorrow. I also have an MRI to sneak in beforehand. It'll be a busy day. I'm really hoping for a visit to the Hockey Hall of Fame on Thursday!

WALL POST

Good morning Facebook world. My schedule has opened up a little for the morning. I have time for extra coffee. I'll be spending a long time in the chemo chair today. I'll tune in with you later. Today was my first shower without help, first time keeping the bandage off, and first time making a medication decision entirely on my own. It's been a red letter day so far.

WALL POST

Good morning everyone. I had a good sleep. I woke up late and was told I'm late for the hospital already. There have been way too many doctors and too much hospital lately. I know breaking my arm is partly my fault, but the rest is cancer's, so I deserve a break. A weekend of camping should just about cover it! Come and rescue me Michelle! I'm going crazy!

WALL POST
FRIDAY, JUNE 29, 2012 AT 2:54 PM

Off to camp 'til Stacey's housewarming on Sunday. Camp is even out of cell range so I am really taking a break. I'll check in, but I'm gone for a few days! Take care of yourselves girls and boys.

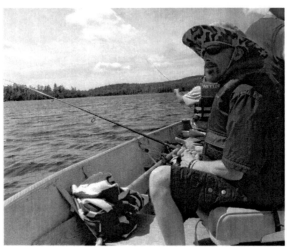

Michael fishing on Canada Day weekend
Photo Courtesy of Michelle Orpel-Stolz

MICHELLE POSTED TO MICHAEL ANTCLIFFE
SATURDAY, JUNE 30, 2012 AT 6:09 PM

Hi everyone, Michael asked me to update you all on his weekend so far. He is having a great time. He even caught some fish! It's been a very relaxing getaway. We'll have fireworks and a band tonight. He will check in with you all tomorrow. Hope everyone has a great weekend and Happy Canada Day!

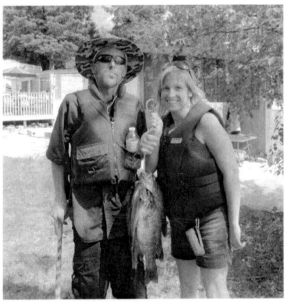

Michael and Michelle at camp
Photo Courtesy of Michelle Orpel-Stolz

STACEY POSTED TO MICHAEL ANTCLIFFE
Monday, July 2, 2012 at 10:35 PM

Just a quick update: I saw Michael tonight and he's alive and well, but he took a bit of a spill last night and is hurting. Georgina, I forgot to give him your cake yesterday, but I had the chance to bring it with me when I went by tonight. I had some of mine and it is yummeh!

WALL POST
Wednesday, July 4, 2012 at 12:10 AM

Good night from la la land guys!

STACEY POSTED TO MICHAEL ANTCLIFFE
THURSDAY, JULY 5, 2012 AT 7:11 PM

Just so you guys know, Michael is still around; he's just doing a lot of resting. I'm not sure if he's reading all of the messages on here, but the sheer number and content is very heartwarming. If I hear that anything changes, I'll be sure to let you all know. I'm not family, so I can't guarantee that I'll hear or that I'll be in the loop. I'm trying to give Michael and his family their privacy, which is why I didn't probe for details about his fall on Sunday night. He didn't break anything and the next day he looked like he was in a bit less pain. We all have to try to curb our concern and curiosity and let Michael step out of the public eye for a bit if that's what he needs right now. That doesn't mean you should stop your well-wishes. It's amazing to see how many people have been brought together by this one exceptional man and what a big family we've become.

WALL POST

Good night, love you all.

WALL POST
SATURDAY, JULY 7, 2012 AT 9:56 PM

Well hello. I'm fine. It's been a rough week with a throat infection. Still alive and well. Friends to visit!

WALL POST
MONDAY, JULY 9, 2012 AT 6:59 PM

Who still reads despite my lack of updates?

WALL POST
MONDAY, JULY 9, 2012 AT 7:48 PM

I feel better today than yesterday. Better than the day before, no idea what the big picture is?

WALL POST
TUESDAY, JULY 10, 2012 AT 8:58 PM

Much of life is getting figured out.

STACEY POSTED TO MICHAEL ANTCLIFFE
TUESDAY, JULY 17, 2012 AT 3:53 PM

I talked to Michael a little while ago and he said I should tell you all that he's still alive. He's having a hard time getting on Facebook. He's having a hard time with texts, too. Phone is a bit better.

WALL POST
TUESDAY, JULY 17, 2012 AT 5:26 PM

Wow, I have 5,000 friends. Thanks everyone for the support, looking forward to seeing more of you in the future. For those I can't add, you can join the *I owe Michael Antcliffe $10* page.

MICHELLE POSTED TO MICHAEL ANTCLIFFE
Friday, July 20, 2012 at 4:24 PM

Michael asked me to update you all on what's been going on. Here's what he would like to say:

Had a rough couple of days with balance and speaking, so I was in the hospital. I'm home now and doing a little better. I'm still a bit of a muppet head. Thank you to all of my 5,000 friends.

STACEY POSTED TO MICHAEL ANTCLIFFE
Sunday, July 22, 2012 at 7:54 PM

Hey folks! I visited with Michael last night and he was still as stubborn as ever. The main reason he's not updating Facebook often is that his vision really isn't good enough to allow him on here. I try to read him your comments and help him with an update when I'm visiting, but please don't worry if he doesn't post for a few days. Michael has been getting a lot of help and is doing all right.

DANIELLE POSTED TO MICHAEL ANTCLIFFE
MONDAY, JULY 23, 2012 AT 7:23 PM

Hey everyone, I'm here visiting with Michael. He is alive and well; his dad and mom are taking really good care of him. Michael says hello to all. He thanks everyone for all the love and support. He really appreciates the ongoing well-wishes.

STACEY POSTED TO MICHAEL ANTCLIFFE
TUESDAY, JULY 24, 2012 AT 6:54 PM

Hello all! I had a long visit with Michael today and he was sitting up and watching TV. We had some great conversation — boy can that man make me smile. I got a few good smiles out of him, too, even though today was a bit painful. He asked me to update you and when I asked him what he wanted me to say, he said, "Tell them what you see." I had a hard time seeing beyond his stubbornness and his smile. He told me today that apparently I'm not the only one who calls him stubborn — go figure! He also said it was about time he was getting back on his feet. I told him he had 5,000 people sending him the strength to do so.

MICHELLE POSTED TO MICHAEL ANTCLIFFE
WEDNESDAY, JULY 25, 2012 AT 4:03 PM

Hi everyone. I'm here with Michael and just wanted to update you all with some words from Michael:

I'm still a muppet head and I have no idea what I'm watching on TV. A male nurse is heading over soon to help me shower for the first time . . . at least I think it's a male nurse, lol. Have a good day and night everyone. Love you all. Take it easy.

Michael is in good spirits and laughing and smiling today. Your support helps :) Thank you.

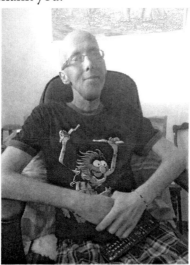

Michael being a muppet head
Photo Courtesy of Michelle Orpel-Stolz

MICHELLE POSTED TO MICHAEL ANTCLIFFE

FRIDAY, JULY 27, 2012 AT 3:42 PM

Hey everyone. I'm here with Michael and just wanted to write an update for him in his own words:

I'm happy that Michelle is here and brought my little friends Maddi and Alex to visit and that Julie came, too. I'm enjoying a coffee and doughnut. Family is here as well, so it's been a busy afternoon, but I'm loving it. Have a great day everyone. Take it easy. Love you all.

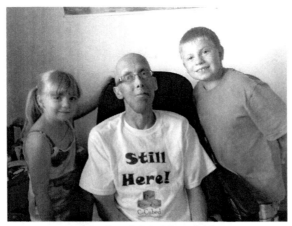

Michael with Maddi and Alex
Photo Courtesy of Michelle Orpel-Stolz

STACEY POSTED TO MICHAEL ANTCLIFFE
TUESDAY, JULY 31, 2012 AT 3:26 PM

Good afternoon everyone! Kevin Chlebovec and I visited with Michael today, and he told me to tell you all that he was awake and still here. Kevin is the other editor/publisher for Michael's book (and lives in Toronto), so it was really nice that he finally got to meet the man in person. I've been on Facebook and accepted more friend requests, so we're back up to 5,000. While I was there, Michael enjoyed some doughnuts and we had a nice talk about unions and teaching and a variety of other non-cancer-related stuff. I forgot his milkshake today, but that was all right because his uncle had just brought him coffee and doughnuts. I passed on some gentle hugs for everyone.

MICHELLE POSTED TO MICHAEL ANTCLIFFE
Tuesday, July 31, 2012 at 3:39 PM

Hey everyone I'm here with Michael with another update in his words:

Hello, still alive . . . how is everyone? Glad to still be here. Happy that I can get people to update Facebook for me. I'm still a muppet head. Have a great day everyone. Love you all.

MICHELLE POSTED TO MICHAEL ANTCLIFFE
SATURDAY, AUGUST 4, 2012 AT 3:48 PM

Hey everyone here's another update in Michael's own words:

Hey everyone! I'm still alive and looking forward to my bath with a gorgeous nurse. :) Obviously, I have my own private nurse. Hope everyone is having a good weekend. Please take care of each other. Thanks again for being here. Love you all.

I read all the posts from everyone to Michael as well. Have a great day everyone.

MICHELLE POSTED TO MICHAEL ANTCLIFFE
TUESDAY, AUGUST 7, 2012 AT 10:10 PM

Hi everyone . . . just letting you know that Michael says hi to everyone and that he's still smiling. He is extra tired today so I said I would update for him and he could update in his words maybe tomorrow if he isn't too tired. Take care everyone and have a great evening.

FROM CANDICE
Sunday, August 19, 2012

Ok kid . . . here goes . . .

You'll Never Guess Who casually walked into my life a year-and-a-half ago.

You'll Never Guess Who, in such a short time, became an integral part of my heart and therefore my family.

You'll Never Guess Who taught me more about myself than I actually realized then, and now for that matter.

You'll Never Guess Who held my hand during one of the toughest times in my life, and told me that I could do it no matter what, and that I could make the difference without actually being at my side.

You'll Never Guess Who asked me to be a part of your first Relay for Life team and make total strangers into family members.

You'll Never Guess Who has inspired me, as well as thousands of others, to do everything and anything I can to carry your legacy from here on out and keep on keeping on with your dream.

You'll Never Guess Who, in just months, completely changed my world and has made me a better person for it.

You'll Never Guess Who will *never* leave my heart and soul, even though you took a piece of it with you yesterday.

You'll Never Guess Who is my favourite kid on this planet, this side or not . . .

That, my friend, is *you*.

Thank you will never be enough. I'm so glad I got to be a part of your life and was able to tell you those words time and time again.

My heart just aches for Alan and Mary, and the rest of the Antcliffe clan, as well as the family you've created within us, your Relay for Life team. You will always be our fearless team captain and, if I may promise, we will do everything we can to continue to Remember, Fight Back, and Celebrate for your legacy.

FROM MICHELLE
Tuesday, September 18, 2012

I still remember the day you told me that you were dying of cancer. The words were so heavy and unimaginable. I remember thinking *this isn't real.* Yes, obviously I knew cancer existed and how very deadly and unforgiving the disease could be, but I had been *fortunate* enough to know only one person close to me that had been taken by cancer. The fact that it was you sitting with me, eating ice cream, the sun shining . . . it all seemed so unreal. I had known you since my early teens, and hearing the details of the road you were going to face rocked me to my very core. I remember thinking *Michael Antcliffe . . . dying? How could this be?* I was angry, scared, and overwhelmed. So many emotions went through me as you told me. I thought *this is so unfair, he's too young.* Then I realized that you seemed so calm, so strong, so determined to fight with everything you had to the very end. You vowed to make a difference — to take something so horrible and try and make something amazing come out of it.

I then had the amazing privilege to be your friend — to be by your side when you needed me. You were so strong and so damn stubborn (lol). You wanted to do things for yourself, even if it was a struggle. I admired your spirit and determination to not let cancer take any more from you than you were willing to allow. You remained standing when most people would have been brought to their knees, and you always kept your humour and your smile.

I remember how much fun we all had when we went to camp. We

were able to check everything off your bucket list and the fact that I was able to give that to you makes me very happy. We didn't let cancer follow us out there. We had a weekend of as much normalcy as circumstances would allow. There were no doctors, no appointments, nothing but relaxing and having fun. We had so many laughs that weekend and met so many new people that you touched with your courage and strength. We fished, had campfires, watched amazing fireworks on the beach, admired a sunset, had a fish fry, and you got to have the memories that kept you smiling when things got rougher for you. And out of that weekend you got to have your own fish story (I hope by now when you're telling it you are up to ten huge fish, lol). But even with all you were dealing with, you never stopped being concerned for others.

I am so very honoured to have known you when you were young, as well as when you were an early adult. I also had the privilege of watching the courageous and determined man that took what life had dealt him and tried to make every second he had left worth something. You always told people to stop and realize how short life can be and to live every moment like it may be your last. You were always there to give advice or just to listen if anyone needed your ear, even with all you had on your plate. I don't know of too many people who could have done as amazingly with what they were dealt and not instead become angry, bitter, and withdrawn. You remained smiling, laughing, joking, caring, and compassionate no matter what happened to you.

Then you allowed so many people to follow you on your very personal journey. You were so open and honest about what you were thinking, feeling, and going through both physically and emotionally. That, to me, took so much courage — to allow your pain and scary journey to be exposed to people in in the hope that you would make a difference to others that cancer would touch. I admire and respect you for all you have done and all the lives and hearts you touched with your story and your brave journey.

You made me laugh. Seeing your courage, strength and

determination to help others changed me for the better. I often wondered how you kept that smile on your face every time I saw you. How did you keep smiling in spite of everything? You touched so many people and changed so many lives. I hope you are looking down on us, surrounded by pretty women and all the ice cream you can eat, smiling at the difference you have made. This is all because of you, muppet. It's all because you wanted to help others. I remember you telling me "I know cancer will win this war, but I will make sure I give it the biggest fight it's ever seen right 'til the very end." You were determined to get in a few good shots before you went down. And, my friend, you fought the most amazing battle ever. You are one of the most amazing people I have ever met.

I thank you for letting me be a part of your life, for allowing me to give you strength when you needed it, for letting me pick you up when you were weak, for allowing me to make you smile and laugh when you forgot how, and most of all I thank you for all you have given me in return. Your friendship was such a blessing and something I will miss for the rest of my life. I miss your laugh, your smile, your sense of humour, but most of all just talking to you. You will forever be my muppet head.

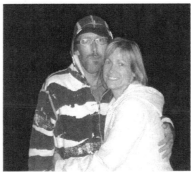

Michael and Michelle
Photo Courtesy of Michelle Orpel-Stolz

AFTERWORD

We have come to the end of Michael's fight with cancer but not to the end of his journey. I mentioned in the foreword that I have put this book together for Michael three times now. Each time has been a very different experience for me.

The first time, I didn't really know Michael, but the countless times that I went through his notes and his wall gave me an insight to his character that made our first in-person meeting very surreal. He would start to tell me a story about something that I had already read about on Facebook, and he would discover that this stranger knew more about him than he knew about her. Once I pointed that out to him, however, he seemed to look at it as a challenge and quickly learned a lot about me, my family, and my life. He always asked how my teenage daughter was doing, and one of my favourite last memories was the last time my two-year-old son visited with him and how Michael's eyes lit up and he said "Danny!" in such a happy voice. One of our most treasured possessions now is the "pimp stick" that Michael broke before leaving on his road trip. After Michael died, his father cut it down, put the top on the smaller piece, and gave the "mini pimp stick" to my son.

The second time I put this book together was before his Memorial Wake that we held in his honour on October 5, 2012. This time, the book contained not only the notes from the time before I really got to know Mike, but also the experiences that I had shared with him. It was an incredibly painful but cathartic process. I am very happy to say that we raised over $10,000.00 at his wake and that all the money went to help people with cancer.

This time, I'm putting Michael's words together to share with the entire world. Michael's dream was to raise a million dollars to help people with cancer, and I have vowed to see that happen in my lifetime. This book is only one of the instruments we're using to make his dream a reality, but it's one of the easiest to track. Instead of paying royalties to his family, Michael's publisher is giving an enormous 90% royalty to the Canadian Cancer Society in Michael's name. How much this truly amounts to depends on the readers. If you've read to this point and Michael's words have touched you, please consider buying a copy for a friend, for your local cancer clinic, or for your local library. Split Tree Publishing is also offering **Hope is my Wingman** to cancer-related charities and non-profits at a steep discount for use either as a tool to help the people they work with or as a means of fundraising.

Michael Antcliffe was a very special man. He found himself faced with death and decided to do something truly inspirational. He didn't leave behind a wife or children, but he left behind hope and a dream. We can either move forward, carrying Michael's message in our hearts and living each day as if it were our last, or continue on with the status-quo, being more caught up with the unimportant details and missing out on the best that life has to offer. In the end, it's your choice.

ABOUT THE AUTHOR

Michael Jack Antcliffe was born May 13th 1975 in the old McKeller Hospital in Thunder Bay, Ontario, Canada. The youngest of three children (siblings Christopher and Jennifer) in a working-class family, Michael spent his early years raised by his parents, Alan and Mary, in a country setting in the township of Scoble, a short distance southeast of the city of Thunder Bay. He enjoyed a childhood that inspired a love of nature and the outdoors. Michael moved back into the city in time to attend Sir Winston Churchill High School and continued his education at the University of Manitoba, where he stayed and worked as a Youth Care Worker at Jessie Home Inc., for five years following the completion of university. Missing his family, Michael returned to his home town and began earning his way doing home renovations and construction, eventually finding employment with a university friend at First Class Finishing. Always choosing to keep life simple and concentrating on time spent with friends and loved ones, Michael continued to follow this philosophy after being afflicted with malignant melanoma and forced onto disability.

During the last year and a half of his life, Michael explored fundraising avenues and sought to improve the lives of those stricken by cancer whose fight each day is simply to reach the next. He made the most of his time, choosing to spend it with family and friends. Michael's siblings, Christopher and Jennifer still live in Thunder Bay, along with their parents.

Michael Jack Antcliffe passed away on August 18th 2012 at the age of 37. He will never be forgotten.